Ann Newman

The Psychiatric Nurse
As A Family Therapist

THE PSYCHIATRIC NURSE AS A FAMILY THERAPIST

Edited by
Shirley Smoyak
Rutgers University
College of Nursing

A Wiley Biomedical-Health Publication
JOHN WILEY & SONS, INC.
New York   London   Sydney   Toronto

To:
My Partner-in-Parenting, Colleague, Lover,
Supporter, Confidante, Critic, Sharer-in-Fun,
All of Whom Are Named, **Neil**

Library of Congress Cataloging in Publication Data:

Main entry under title:

The Psychiatric nurse as a family therapist.

 Selected papers from a series of family therapy workshops held at the University of New Mexico, Albuquerque.
 Includes bibliographical references.
 1. Family psychotherapy—Congresses. 2. Psychiatric nursing—Congresses. I. Smoyak, Shirley.
[DNLM: 1. Family therapy. 2. Psychiatric nursing. WY160 S666p]
RC488.5.P78   616.8'915   75-5813
ISBN 0-471-80770-2

Printed in the United States of America

10 9 8 7 6 5 4 3 2 1

Foreword

New winds are blowing in the health field. No longer is illness viewed solely as a dysfunction of a body part or disturbance of a person in isolation from others. There is a new view: behavior formerly labeled "sick" is instead both a signal and a function of a disturbance in an ongoing system. The most vigorous debates and investigations are now going forward on this development, particularly in its application in regard to family therapy. Nurses participate in this effort.

There are, of course, many reasons for the emerging shift toward viewing illness as a systems phenomenon instead of as an intrapersonal one. Roethlesburger's classic studies at Western Electric indicated the interpersonal influence that one employee could have on the productivity of other workers. Grinker's work during World War II identified as a system effect that some battalion commanders had fewer psychiatric casualties among men in their units than did others. The work of Moreno and Sullivan in elucidating theories of interpersonal relations contributed greatly toward stimulation of interest in interpersonal networks as seen in family and other social systems. These few examples suggest that illness seen as a system phenomenon is an idea whose time has arrived.

In nursing, intrapersonal theories and "descriptive psychiatry" provided explanations that were predominant in basic curricula until the Mental Health Act of 1946 was passed. This act provided funds that aided the development of graduate education in psychiatric nursing. Directors of graduate programs, which by 1952 were supported only at the master's-degree level, were dissatisfied with the limitations placed on nursing practice by descriptive or within-person explanations of the behavior of patients seen in nursing situations. Explanations of behavior of people in groups, reported in social science literature, and theories explanatory of interpersonal relations, particularly Sullivan's work, were seen as fresh sources for generating more viable nursing practices that would benefit patients.

By 1948 the emphasis was on the study of one-to-one, nurse-patient relationships since it was recognized early that the evocative influence of the patient's behavior on the nurse had to be identified, understood, and shifted into new directions. Nurse counseling and nurse psychotherapeutic interviewing derived from this emphasis and quickly filtered down from graduate to basic nursing education programs as a curriculum objective. Moreover, by 1956, clinical workshops from one to six weeks duration began to be offered across the nation to any registered nurse who attended for her to learn psychotherapeutic interviewing. A major insight, however, generated by the rapid acceptance of the study of nurse-patient relationships was recognition of the *nurse as an agent and primary instrument* of change in patients through the practice of psychiatric nursing.

Group approaches in psychiatric nursing practice were dictated largely, although not exclusively, by the economics of health care; in 1952 over 54 percent of all hospital beds available in the United States were for psychiatric patients. Practitioners in all of the professional disciplines — psychiatrists, psychologists, psychiatric nurses, and psychiatric social workers — were in short supply. While individual psychotherapy for a few patients could be justified on the basis of continuing, in-depth study of particular psychiatric phenomena or because of unusual circumstances of a patient, it was considered to be a luxury approach. The demand was to expose many more patients to the potential benefits of various modalities of group work — remotivation, ward government, occupational and recreational groups, and group psychotherapy. Thus nurses, with their high commitment to the improvement of health of patients, also began to study and test theories and methods of group work of various kinds.

It was a step forward for nurses to recognize the family of a hospitalized patient as a particular kind of group and to begin to explore the possibilities of family therapy as an aspect of psychiatric nursing practice. Perhaps more than in any other discipline, nurses employed in psychiatric facilities did observe that interactions between inpatients and their family visitors were problematic. In the late 1940s many attempts were made to meet with groups of families, the expectation being that they could be helped to understand and thus to tolerate, if not to help remedy, the difficulties of members of their families who were hospitalized in psychiatric facilities.

In 1956 the Graduate Program in Psychiatric Nursing at Rutgers[1] included a course called Mental Health in Public Health. In this course various approaches to work with families having identified psychiatric patients were tried, and from this effort a psychiatric nursing form of family therapy was evolved. By 1967 the theory and practice of family therapy were clearly identified, and its beneficial effects sufficiently evident to test a more widespread dissemination to practicing nurses. Dr. Reina Hall, then Dean of Nursing at the University of New Mexico, Albuquerque, obtained a grant[2] that supported a one-month family therapy workshop each year for a five-year period. In each workshop

[1]The College of Nursing and Graduate School, Rutgers, The State University of New Jersey, New Brunswick, New Jersey 08903.
[2]P.H.S. grant number MH 11349-01-05.

group there were 12 students and three faculty members.[3] The aims of the workshop were to test the feasibility of teaching family therapy to registered nurses on a short-course basis and to establish the criteria for admission that would ensure a successful educative experience for the nurses.[4]

The selections in this book were initially prepared by the students in these workshops and were based on their direct clinical work with troubled families. This work documents the readiness and ability of registered nurses to participate with their colleagues in other disciplines in the health care field and in the continuing search for effective methods of intervention.

In the 25 years since the Mental Health Act of 1946 was passed nurses have used the small portion of these funds allocated for nursing programs to enrich the practice of nursing in the interest of enlarging the benefits for the public. One aspect of such practice by nurses is family therapy. It is a form of problem solving that holds great promise. The family therapist initiates changes in a family system by engaging each family member in examining the network of relations and pattern integrations in which each is a participant and by testing out new behaviors. Thus, disturbance in an ongoing family system is recognized, and it becomes the focus for family therapy.

Hildegard E. Peplau, R.N., Ed.D.

---

[3]Dr. Hildegard E. Peplau (1968-1969), Dr. Shirley Smoyak (1968-1972) Dr. William E. Field Jr. (1968-1972), and Dr. Grayce Sills (1970-1972).
[4]A report has been prepared.

Preface

Ten years ago, a psychiatric nurse was not expected to be a family therapist. Times are changing, however. Today, clinical specialists in psychiatric nursing are expected to have the necessary skills to be able to conduct family therapy without supervision. Other psychiatric nurses who work in family-centered agencies are also finding it necessary to acquire these skills and are functioning as therapists under the supervision of master's or doctoral-level nurses or clinicians from other disciplines, such as psychiatry, psychology, or social work. Since theories concerning family dynamics are relatively new, as are the associated techniques and strategies for therapeutic work, practicing nurses must learn both by either returning to school or finding suitable continuing education opportunities.

Historically, nurses recognized the relevance of families, even when a particular person in the family was designated as "The Patient." Nurses knew that, in order to understand and to intervene therapeutically in a pathological situation, the variable of family dynamics was a crucial one. Most undergraduate curricula in nursing have some segment that focuses on dynamics of family concepts. Only some schools, however, introduce the student to family therapy. The situation then is one in which the practitioner knows only too well how important and crucial family dynamics are but where students still lack adequate preparation to practice effectively.

The study of families as systems departs radically from the historical trend of psychiatry and psychology where the focus has been predominately on intrapsychic processes and where often the family has been viewed as disruptive, irrelevant, or benign. The new view is that symptoms are not intrapsychically produced but are signals of system or family distress. Mental illness is a family, not an individual, phenomenon. One can have appendicitis by himself, but he cannot be paranoid, suicidal, or schizophrenic by himself. No competing view of mental illness, be it biological-genetic, chemical, or psychoanalytic, has established itself beyond reasonable doubt. The systems approach is both logical and verifiable by clinical data.

If nurses are to develop their expertise in working therapeutically with troubled families, they need to begin to identify recurrent family dynamics that lead to disruption, states of crisis, or malfunctioning of individual members. The current literature is expanding with hunches and clinical instances of dynamics and intervention tactics. The field, however, is in its infancy as far as categorization or systemization of clinical phenomena and therapeutic strategies is concerned. There is no consensus of a classification of family pathology. There is no agreement about how family data ought to be recorded. In fact, there is no format, manual or computer based, for recording family dynamics and problems. Several large anthologies and review books on the family have been published in the last five years. These provide an accurate overview of what still must be learned.

Since human beings are socialized within family systems to play their future societal roles, it is necessary to seek an understanding of the various styles and workings of these intricate systems as they affect the cognitive and emotional development of their members. An individual-patient approach yields very different outcomes than a family approach because the basic premises are different and influence the practitioners' viewpoint markedly. Jay Haley illustrates this change of view very aptly.

"Over the last few decades there has been a breakdown of the idea that the individual is the unit of study for the proper study of man. This has been happening in a variety of fields, but in psychiatry there are more immediate practical consequences. The most extreme issue has arisen in regard to the schizophrenic. It was once assumed that of all people we needed to be least concerned about the context of living of the schizophrenic because he was withdrawn from reality and therefore his reality situation was irrelevant. This seems hard to believe now, but it was once flatly assumed. Then about the 1940s people began to discover and talk about the mothers of schizophrenics. It has been known for a long time that schizophrenics had mothers, but they appeared irrelevant because of the nature of schizophrenia and because the mothers in many cases seemed like nice people and the patient was behaving in such a screwy way that she couldn't possibly have anything to do with it. At first it was suggested that the mother must have done something back in infancy that scarred this patient in some way so that now he was just a walking thing. This seemed interesting, but it was rather unimportant because it happened years ago. However, some people began to suggest that the mother was currently (emphasis mine) *doing something which kept the schizophrenic behaving like a schizophrenic. This was a very different kind of idea. The question became, 'Is this mother dealing with this child differently from the way a mother deals with her normal child.' I think this question is a major event of this century."* [1]

[1] Jay Haley, "The Family Structure and its Importance to the Individual," *The Quarterly of Camarillo,* Vol. 2, No. 2, May, 1966, pp. 5–6.

As soon as one begins to work on this very large task of studying recurring family dynamics that lead to some kind of system disturbance, it becomes obvious that one of the confounding problems is our language. Our present terminology for describing human behavior had its origins in the days of intrapsychic psychiatry. The words are largely descriptive of individual behavior or individual processes, rather than interpersonal or system processes. Consider, for instance, such concepts as anxiety, frustration, ambivalence, conflict, aggression, dominance, and submission. When the study of human behavior began to move from a "within-self" view to an interpersonal one, the age of the hyphen was born. Thus, clinicians and theorists spoke of dominance-submission, masochism-sadism, aggressive-passive, and so on. It was not too difficult to follow the train of thought or logic as the hyphen was used. There was even an attempt to describe the relationship per se, instead of the actors. Empathy would be an example of such an interpersonal concept. However, the problem of language is much greater when a systems model is used. Of course, still another hyphen might be added, and at least a triangular process could be described, but who was doing what would not be specified. Single-word concepts do not seem to be able to adequately handle the conceptual traffic that systems analysis requires. For instance, equilibrium is a systems concept, but no one is quite sure to what it refers. An observer can sometimes say that a particular system is in "disequilibrium," but having said that, he has not described how it got that way. The present trend, in deriving an adequate language for this new approach, seems to be the use of phrases such as "coalition across generations."

In order to identify recurring family dynamics, the process of interaction among the members must be operationalized. In other words, before naming the dynamic, the specific recurring interaction must be spelled out with utmost clarity. Only after collecting many instances of these repetitious family phenomena can they be examined and analyzed for similarities and differences.

The Family Workshop at the University of New Mexico, Albuquerque, was the first one of its kind in continuing education for nurses. It admitted only those nurses who were motivated toward becoming practicing family therapists. Its goals were to develop clinical practitioners who based their interventions on theory, who were committeed to a constant process of questioning and discovery, and who would communicate their efforts to others in writing. The selections in this book are an outgrowth of the five summers in which the workshop was held.

A total of 61 registered nurses was enrolled in the program during its five-year duration. Twelve trainees were admitted yearly; in one year there was an additional faculty from the University of New Mexico College of Nursing.

Trainees included whites, blacks, and Spanish-speaking individuals. The age range was from 25 to 64, with a mean age of 40. One trainee had a Ph.D., 22 had master's degrees in nursing, and 17 had diplomas in nursing. Virtually all of those with a diploma in nursing had taken additional courses since graduation.

At the time of enrollment in the workshop, 23 were faculty members, 3 were graduate students in nursing, 9 were inservice educators, 1 was an R.N. in a B.S.N. program, 9 were staff nurses, 5 were head nurses in a psychiatric hospital, 4 were supervisors, 4 were directors of nursing, 1 was a nurse therapist in private practice, 1 was a provincial coordinator, and 1 had no position at the time of the workshop. Additionally, 3 were members of religious orders.

A psychiatric nurse who is a family therapist is also doing basic research on the family process. The reason for this, it seems to me, is that at present, no discipline in the behavioral sciences, basic or advanced, has provided sufficiently sound theory and intervention techniques for the practice of family therapy. If the nurse's goal is to be therapeutic in her relationships with families, then first she must discover just which intervention tactics are therapeutic and which ones are not. The only route to that answer is through research. Not *every* nurse-therapist must spend X number of hours in basic research. However, every nurse-therapist must realize what she does not know about family practice and must look for ways to share her data with nurses who are engaged in more active research projects in the area of family dynamics.

I have suggested that the search for understanding in the family field must operationalize recurring family dynamics in order to develop appropriate intervention strategies. The selections in this book reflect that intent. The search for systematization, however, usually has taken a less-dynamic route. There have been several major attempts to provide classification schemes, but these schemes did not focus on the interaction process per se and hence seem to be of limited use by clinical practioners. One approach has been to evolve a classification of crises[2] while another has concentrated on categorizing family functions.[3]

Langsley and his associates developed a tentative listing of the types of family crisis. The list consists of: (1) the "bolt from the blue" crisis; (2) the caretaker crisis; (3) the developmental crisis, and (4) the exacerbation crisis. They conclude, however, that "These categories have not really been satisfactory and most cases seen by the Family Therapy Unit fit into the 'exacerbation' model. To date a typology of crises which adequately

[2]Donald Langsley, et al, "Family Crisis Therapy — Results and Implications," in *Family Process,* Vol. 7, No. 2, September, 1968.

[3]Stephen Fleck, "On Approach to Family Pathology" in *Comprehensive Psychiatry,* Vol. 7, No. 5, October, 1966, pp. 307-320.

deals with the stress and the family is not available. This challenge is a worthy one.''[4]

Fleck states, ''Defining family abnormalities is complex, and the examination and evaluation of family functions or tasks seems the most appropriate approach to determining and outlining family pathology.''[5] The list of family functions he suggests include (1) parental coalition, (2) nurturant tasks, (3) enculturation of the younger generation, (4) emancipation of offspring from the family, and (5) family crises. His approach, then, is to study deficiencies in and deviations from salient family functions and tasks. Although his method is a very logical one, it, too, does not focus on dynamics. Fleck's conclusion is, ''It is not possible at present to establish specific correlation between such defects and clinical psychiatric entities.''[6]

Other efforts at systematization have utilized the ''microscopic'' method, whereby behavior is dissected into microunits for analysis. Bales et. al., at the Harvard Social Relations Laboratories, have been doing this for several years with various kinds of groups. Bachrach recently reported using electronic and computer methods to analyze bits of schizophrenic speech.[7]

In summary, the search for order in the field has ranged from microscopic theories and methods to macroscopic ones. The approach that workshop participants, will illustrate by their selections, is a middleground one. That is, beginning theory neither resorts to very small subbits of communication for analysis, nor does it propose all-inclusive, grand-theory dimensions. Operationalizing family dynamics allows the nurse to generate family theory and to develop intervention strategies. These theories and strategies need testing for cross-cultural relevance. So far, very little has been done in the area of ethnic differences among families and how these affect interaction mechanisms. The data that are available are largely descriptive and not specifically addressed to family therapy issues.[8]

The orientation-to-family-therapy format alluded to in several of the readings was developed from my experience in working with families from several different agencies over a number of years. Right now I make it a point, and ask students to do the same in the first session, to specify three major areas: (1) assurances, (2) ''truths,'' and (3) directions. Assur-

[4]Langsley, *op. cit.* p. 157.
[5]Fleck, *op. cit.* pp. 307–308.
[6]*Ibid,* p. 319.
[7]A. J. Bachrach, ''Structural Analysis of Schizophrenic Speech: Sound Spectographic Data,'' Paper presented at Conference on Schizophrenia, Eastern Psychiatric Research Association, Inc., New York, November 14, 1968.
[8]For instance, Oscar Lewis' work with Mexican and Puerto Rican families and Beatrice Whiting's *Six Cultures.*

ances include statements by the nurse concerning what is likely to happen in any family session. The members are told that nothing more disruptive or damaging will happen as a result of talking together. Words such as, "You all have already experienced tremendous upsets and upheavals. What goes on with me, here, won't be any worse. In fact, very shortly, the whole business will seem clearer." This is to allay the fears that some families seem to have about terrible, uncontrollable monsters being raised in the process of therapy.

"Truths" include statements by the nurse about how systems work. For instance, "Symptoms are signals; they are ways that people have for telling each other, without words, that something is wrong." I also tell the members to expect temporary disruption in their usual interaction patterns that result when one member begins to define himself a bit differently. The family is told that each affects the other and that no one ever operates in a social vacuum.

Directions include suggestions from the nurse on how they are to proceed with the work. Nurses define themselves *not* as medical model healers but as systems analysts who are present and available for consultation. The family is told to say their thoughts "out loud" and to begin with the current difficulty.

Shirley Smoyak

Acknowledgments

My thanks go to the following individuals: Hildegard E. Peplau for giving me the idea of the workshop, for her encouragement of students, and for being a model as a teacher and clinician. To Reina Hall, ex-Dean, for writing and negotiating for the USPHS-HEW grant that funded the workshop. To B. Louise Murray, Dean, School of Nursing, for her continued support. To Cosma Reinhart and Judy Maurin, faculty members and workshop participants, School of Nursing, University of New Mexico, who served as coordinators for agency contacts.

To those agencies that served as referring agencies over the five years and for their cooperation in allowing students to interview families in their caseloads — in some instances for use of one-way vision rooms and television equipment, were the following:

1. Child Guidance Center: This is a private agency that referred families to the workshop during the years.

2. Bernalillo County Mental Health Center. This is a community mental health facility associated with the UNM Medical School, Department of Psychiatry and University Hospital. This agency participated all five years by providing families for workshop trainees. Families were referred from the Inpatient Unit, the Community Teams, the Outpatient Unit, and the Adolescent Program, and the Narcotic Addict Rehabilitation Program.

3. Nazareth Hospital. This is a private psychiatric hospital located approximately 10 miles from the center of the city. In the first year families were selected from this institution; however, in the remaining years only housing and classroom facilities were used.

4. Programs for Children. This program, a division of the Bernalillo County Mental Health Center, was a participating agency during the fourth and fifth years. The program offers services to families of preschool emotionally disturbed children, multiply handicapped children, and emotionally disturbed retarded children.

5. Veterans' Administration Hospital: This agency also participated all five years. Families were referred from the Day Treatment Center, Inpatient Unit, and Mental Hygiene programs of this agency.

To Grayce Sills, Ph.D., William Field, Ph.D., and other faculty for the workshop who listened to ideas, helped formulate content, and provided beginning editing.

Shirley Smoyak

Table of Contents

Contributors

Chapter   **Author**

1.   Grayce Sills, R.N.

Professor and Program Director, Graduate Program in Psychiatric-Mental Health Nursing, The Ohio State University. Vice-President, Board of Trustees, Southwest Area Community Mental Health Center, Columbus, Ohio

2.   Imelda Wiltz Clements, R.N.

Consultant in Family Therapy, Veterans' Administration Hospital, Murphreesboro, Tennessee. Doctoral Candidate, Peabody College

      Diane Buchanan, R.N., M.S.

Clinical Specialist, Parkview Hospital, Nashville, Tennessee

3.   Nellie M. Rodgers, R.N.

Coordinator of Supportive Living Services, North De Kalb Community Mental Health Center, Atlanta, Georgia

4.   Barbara Croddy, R.N.

Training Consultant for River Region Mental Health-Mental Retardation Services, Louisville, Kentucky.

5.   Marilyn A. Garin, R.N.

Baccalaureate in Nursing candidate, Granite City, Illinois

6.   Pamela Herriott, R.N.

Psychiatric Nurse In-Service Instructor, North Carolina Memorial Hospital, Chapel Hill, North Carolina

7.   Sharon Pecha, R.N.

Nursing Coordinator, Programs for Children, Bernalillo County Mental Health and Mental Retardation Center, Albuquerque, New Mexico

8.   Gwen Gorman, R.N.

Assistant Professor, University of New Mexico (on leave). Masters' Candidate, Arizona State University, Community Health Masters' Program, Tempe, Arizona

9.   Jeannine Dunwell, R.N.

Assistant Professor, University of Hawaii, School of Nursing, Hawaii

10.   Helen Brandt Battiste, R.N.

Formerly, In-patient Nursing Supervisor, Bernalillo County Mental Health Center, Albuquerque, New Mexico

11.   Ida Silver, R.N.

Assistant Professor, C. W. Post College, Greenvale, Long Island, New York

12.   Sister M. Rosalie Whalen, R.N.

Instructor of Psychiatric Nursing, Area I Vocational-Technical School, Dubuque, Iowa

13.   Aurelia Sue Kennedy, R.N.

Licensed Marriage, Family, Child Counselor, Saratoga, California. Private practice.

14.   Jo Ann McKay, R.N.

Private practice in Marriage and Family Counseling, San Francisco Bay Area. Special focus on women.

15.   Harriett E. Goodspeed, R.N.

Formerly, Assistant Professor, Fairleigh Dickinson University, Rutherford, New Jersey

16.   Joella H. Rand, R.N.

Associate Professor, Alfred University, Willard, New York. Urban Division Chairperson.

17.   Ruth Hunt Roberts, R.N.

Head Nurse, Alcoholic Rehabilitation Program, Veterans' Administration Hospital, Albuquerque, New Mexico.

18.   Patricia Fitzpatrick, R.N.

Instructor, Graduate Program in Psychiatric-Mental Health Nursing, University of Illinois, College of Nursing, Chicago, Illinois

19.   Josephine Vander Meer, R.N.

Doctoral Candidate, University of New Mexico, Department of Guidance and Counseling — College of Education, Albuquerque, New Mexico

20.   Lois Jean Plachecki, R.N.

Formerly, Psychiatric Staff Nurse, Nazareth Psychiatric Hospital, Albuquerque, New Mexico

21.   Mary Jane Carter, R.N.

School Nurse, Albuquerque Public School System, Cibola High School, Albuquerque, New Mexico

22.   Sally E. Harris, R.N.

Public Health Nurse I, Wake County Health Department, Wake County, North Carolina

23.   Loretta M. Birckhead, R.N.

Doctoral Candidate, Doctor of Nursing Science Program, Boston University, Boston, Massachusetts

24.   Judith T. Maurin, R.N.

Doctoral Candidate, University of Missouri, Columbia, Missouri

25.   Letha Lierman, R.N.

Assistant Professor, University of Nevada at Reno, Orvis School of Nursing, Reno, Nevada

Introducing Families
to Family Therapy

Shirley Smoyak

Families enter into a therapeutic process or relationship for a variety of reasons. The most frequent reasons will be listed and examples given, before proceding to a discussion of family orientation.

1. They may have come to the self-generated conclusion that an outside source of help is needed.

Tension in the marital relationship or in the area of parental concerns may be so great — the discomfort felt by one or more family members may be so severe — that the entire family, or one of its members as primary speaker, seeks out help. The discomforts usually include varying degrees of anxiety (occasionally panic episodes), psychosomatic symptoms, asocial or antisocial behavior, psychotic behavior, failures at school or work, and so on.

2. The family may have been pushed or shoved, as it were, by another sector of society, toward seeking help for its problems. The family may not necessarily agree with the societal sector that it has a problem. School systems, welfare boards, parole officers, judges — all of these, from time to time, act to move the family into therapy. In some communities, for instance, it has become fairly common practice for juvenile officers and judges to consult with and to refer to community mental health agencies' personnel.

3. Families may intend to label one of their members as sick, in order to hospitalize, remove from power, or remove the member as a threat. The mental health professional, then, is sought as a validator of the family's idea and not a change agent. One family, for instance, sought to label an adopted son as schizophrenic so that he could be "hospitalized and given proper care" when a natural son was born to the parents.

4. The total family may enter therapy in order to understand what they perceive as the problematic behavior of one member. This so-called problem member may or may not go along with this motive. Sometimes this member actively agrees that he or she, is the sole cause of all the distress and that if he or she would change, all would be beautiful. Just as frequently, however, the identified patient may object to this status and come to the family session to plead the case. The former is more likely the case with women and children while the latter instance occurs more often with men and young adults.

5. One or more family members may have been in traditional psychotherapy or in treatment for a physical or psychosomatic illness and been referred by the physician or therapist. Recently I was asked to assess the system dynamics of a couple who had been in traditional therapy for three years. They had entered therapy to find out whether or not they should marry (both had been divorced and both had children) and after three years still did not know. Family therapy provided the arena in which they came to the answer quickly.

Whatever the reason or the circumstances that brings the family to the point of contacting a mental health professional, the following process for orientation and intake is suggested. I have used this process in its present form for about 5 years, evolving roughly after a 10-year period in which various methods were explored by trial and error, supervision of graduate students in various disciplines, and dialogue with colleagues at family therapy conferences. However, the actual process might be modified in given instances, but beginners do find it useful to have some specific steps outlined.

Whatever route the family has taken to enter a therapeutic relationship, the first step for the mental health professional is contacting the family for an appointment. This contact may be made by telephone. However, a home visit might be necessitated as an initial step if there is no telephone in the home and if a nearby relative or neighbor has not offered the use of one.

On the telephone, or in person, tell the family member who you are. Spell your name if there is any possibility that it will be misheard or hard to pronounce. Ask for the family member who made the initial contact or the one who will be responsible for setting up the first appointment. If the person to whom you have been speaking is not the one who will schedule the session, be sure to say and to spell your name when you begin speaking with that person. Take notes during this conversation — important clues will be given regarding *who* thinks there is or is not a problem, who the primary decision maker is, how open or how secret the trouble is, and so on. I have contacted families where a six-year-old has answered the phone, and been aware that a family therapist would be calling. On the other hand, I have spoken with wives who didn't know their husbands had been in contact with an agency, or vice versa.

After identifying yourself by name, say what your discipline is — psychiatry, psychiatric nursing, social work, psychology — and what your *agency title* is — clinician, intern, resident, graduate student, or staff nurse.

Third, tell what information you have on the intake slip or referral form concerning the method of referral and the reason for the request for help. For instance, you might say, "I understand that the child study team at Meadowbrook School recommended a family evaluation for you since Susan's classroom performance does not match the ability she appears to have, measured by tests. Her teacher was also concerned about her frequent tears and fatigue." Wait for the family member to validate this information, correct it, question it, or add to it. Take notes.

Next, say what you will do — which is to use a systems perspective in a family session, to assess or evaluate the presenting problem and plan the next steps. I say something like this: "We have found after working with many, many individuals in a variety of mental health agencies, that when one member is having difficulty, he or she affects everyone else. No one can have a symptom by him or herself. Furthermore, a more accurate way to describe this is that the one who apparently has the symptom or the trouble, is in fact signaling or calling attention to a difficulty that is really a system or family problem. That is why it is very important to have everyone involved or concerned present at this first family session."

This leads you directly into a discussion of who should be there for the family's first session and when it should take place. First sessions generally tend to be scheduled in the evening so that school-children and those who work can attend. Sometimes, when the presenting problem is severe enough (e.g., an acute psychotic episode or an impending hospitalization for depression or somatic complaints), the family will cancel all other obligations and activities and ask to be seen immediately. Everyone who lives in that particular household should be there and also any extended family members who are closely involved. This includes infants, pre-schoolers, school-age children, adults of all ages, boarders, and pets. Those who don't speak (infants, pets) still provide very important data about how that system is organized or disorganized.

The family's home is the logical place for a first visit, and very often is the place of choice for all subsequent therapy. Suggest to the family that they be seen in their own home. It is the rare family who insists on coming to the agency for the session. All last year in my own caseloads and those I supervised, there was only one family who was not seen at home — and in that instance I think it was more the reluctance of the therapist than the family. The advantages of a home visit far outweigh the disadvantages. Among the advantages are gathering data about the family's life-style and place within the community, use of living space within the home, shrines, and cultural artifacts and seeing how anxiety is handled, how the therapist is introduced, what is done about interruptions, and so on. Disadvantages include allocating travel time and, perhaps, a safety factor at night in certain neighborhoods.

Ask for travel directions to the home if you are not certain. And be sure to allow yourself enough time to find the home and be on time for the session.

Tell the family that you will be bringing a tape recorder. The reason for the recorder is to insure that you will have the information accurately when you write your notes for the records.

If another therapist will be accompanying you, say who this will be — a cotherapist, a therapist in training, or a graduate student observer, for example. If this other person will be strictly an observer, I introduce him or her as a "human recorder." Assure the family of the confidentiality of the material they discuss. The records are for professionals only; assure them that they will be asked for their permission before any other agency is given access to the records — including school systems and parole boards.

You will need at least one-and-a-half hours for this first session and probably two. Small families — four persons or less — can generally be handled in one-and-a-half hours. But larger families, or those in crisis situations, take at least two hours. Make sure that you arrive on time, leave on time, and leave the family with a clear idea of what will happen next.

Before ending your telephone or planning contact, have the family member tell you what he or she understands about the time and duration, place, who will be there, and what will happen.

At the beginning of the first visit, all of this orienting material should be repeated. Keep in mind that most of the family members will be anxious in varying degrees — and the higher the anxiety, the less accurate the hearing or understanding of what is being said.

When you arrive at the family's home for this first session (either alone or with the cotherapist or observer) bear in mind that you are the intruder-guest. Resist the urge to take over, to direct the seating, and so on. Wait to be invited. Simply say that the session should occur in a room where everyone can be seated comfortably and hear each other. Then wait to see who decides where to go and how to be seated. Do not be a data wrecker. A data wrecker is a therapist who interferes with systems' dynamics prematurely and hence never knows what the usual pattern or interactions are.

After being directed to a seat or place, adjust the recorder as you repeat the orienting material — who you are and why you came. If someone in the family has never heard his or her voice recorded before, offer to play back some of the tape at the end of the session.

Although I always use a mechanical audiorecorder for family sessions, I find concurrent note taking indispensable. It helps me to keep focused and to prevent the family from using inviting distractions to prevent the analysis of the problem.

I use a legal-size pad — which is the right size for filing and large enough to draw the family tree — that I will discuss shortly.

Ask for the names of all of the people present. I write them on the pad, in a schematic drawing of how they are seated. This is especially useful in families with many members. Be sure you have the correct spelling. Ask each person what he or she would prefer to be called — the way you introduce yourself signals to the family your own preference.

After repeating the basic orienting material, it is time to set some of the ground rules and to lay out the work to be done. The ground rules are few: (1) it is better to make things (thoughts, feelings, hunches) overt than to keep them covert — better out than in; and (2) everyone in a family session has an equal voice but not necessarily an equal vote. The latter is especially important to clarify when there are children present. By clarifying the "voice/not necessarily vote" rule, the therapist reinforces the expectation that all persons will be active in the session. This does not mean, however, that children necessarily have a vote in decisions. It forces the parents, or decision makers, however, to consider the question of at what age, if ever, their children will have a vote in family matters. For some kinds of families — for instance, traditional, Catholic Italians, the answer is "never." A child is a child (meaning he does what parents tell him to do) so long as the parents are alive.

Next, I tell the family how the time will be used during this session. I say it similar to this: "All that I know about you is here on this intake slip. I'll share that information with you in a moment. What I need to know before we can proceed with the work is who exactly you all are, how you got here, and how you are related to each other. So for roughly the first half of this session, I'll ask you specific questions and put the information on this family tree. Now you might be wondering why I want to know about all of you, when apparently just one of you is having some trouble. The reason is that now we know that people can't have symptoms by themselves. They are closely, intimately connected with others — they affect others and are affected by them. Let me give you an example — "

Here I use a systems analogy relevant to the life-style of this particular family. Some examples follow shortly.

Then I say, "For the second half of this session, you all will be invited to say what you think the difficulty is — just how troublesome it is — and what you think is necessary for change to be possible. At the end, I will list my observations for you and suggest what you might plan as your therapeutic program. All of this will probably take about two hours, but I guarantee that you will not be bored. In fact, you will be surprised at how much ground you've covered — things you'll find out about each other that you never knew before, and the time will pass quickly. Before I begin with the who's who piece, let me say just one more thing — and I'll be repeating this from time to time, and that is that I see family therapy as "no fault" therapy. The aim is not to blame — but rather to understand and to *change* when necessary. Families are sometimes leery or a bit nervous about investigating themselves in a therapy program — let me assure you that this will be no worse than the things you've already said and done or (left undone) to each other. Occasionally family members say and do mean, malicious, nasty, hurtful things to each other. The aim here is not to lay blame for these happenings but to figure out a way to prevent their reoccurrence. I will take the responsibility for telling you when you are on a laying-blame beam and help you to get off it — your responsibility is to be open and honest. O.K.? Do we have a contract?"

For however long the family needs — usually not more than 10 minutes or so — I encourage them to raise questions about the introduction or orientation. If they try to say what the difficulty is, I stop them and tell them that I need to have the structure and data first so I can listen more intelligently.

At this point, let me share some systems' analogies that have been used in orienting families to the systems' perspective. The more the analogy embodies the major system principles, the better or more accurate the analogy is. My suggestion is that you listen carefully to the tapes[1] on general systems theory and construct your own analogies for the families with whom you'll be working.

EXAMPLE OF FAMILY SYSTEM ANALOGY
Families and Sopaipillas as Systems by LaRae Peters[2]

"Families are systems made up of many parts which work together according to certain rules that they make for themselves. Any system is made up of a certain combination of parts which are necessary to each other in order to make a whole. When the parts work together, they become something more than each could ever be separately.

[1]Audio cassette tapes available from P-S-F Productions, 603 East Olmos Drive, San Antonio, Texas, 78212.
[2]Ms. Peters was a participant in the U. of New Mexico Family Therapy Workshop in 1972.

"For example, it is possible to make some delicious sopaipillas if you have all of the necessary ingredients, flour, baking powder and water. But until they are properly mixed and prepared, they are just ingredients. A change in any of the ingredients will affect the final product. If corn-meal is used instead of flour, or milk instead of water, the result will be changed. When making dough, it is important to add ingredients in a certain order. Families also come together in a certain order. Two individuals marry and learn to live together, then as children are added to the system, it becomes more complicated so that it is necessary to make different rules to allow the system to function. In dough making, the addition of more water makes it necessary to add more flour, for the quantity of ingredients must be in balance. This works in a similar way in families. For instance, if new members are added, a change must be made in the amount of food obtained and prepared.

"Even properly mixed, the dough cannot become crisp, hollow sopaipillas without oil of the right temperature. Nor can a woman be a mother without a child. If any ingredient is missing, the sopaipillas will be changed. The flour cannot raise by itself.

"If the water is too cool for the sopaipillas to rise, it is not the fault of the water alone, it is also the fact that the other ingredients require water of a certain temperature in order to react well together. In the same way, it is the interaction of the entire family system that needs attention rather than any single member.

"All sopaipillas are somewhat alike and yet when the pieces of dough are dropped into the hot oil, they rise according to the amount of baking powder, the heat of the oil and the thickness of the pieces. All of these factors and others determine what any particular cook's sopaipillas are like. In the same way certain ingredients in family parts make each family somewhat different. Families are made up of many different combinations of members, differences in cultural background, in ways of doing things and in the things they feel are important. Like the sopaipillas all the parts are important and success in the family depends on all the parts working together."

For another family — in which there were members who, by vocation and avocation, were theater people — the putting together of a stage play was used.

I view the first half of an intake session as the gathering of *structural* data and the second half as discovering the *functions* or *system interactions process* (if that term is more comfortable for you). In actual practice, it is not possible to separate structure from function, but it is helpful to keep in mind that a systems analysis requires two different dimensions: what the parts are and how they are related; these are the significant categories.

You need to develop your own particular style of eliciting the structural data about a family. This is the way I do it.

On the pad, halfway down the page, I draw two circles, connecting them with a line. (This is if there are a mother and father or husband and wife in the particular constellation — if there is only one primary adult — a mother, for instance, I draw one circle and a dotted line to another dotted circle to designate the biological father of the children.) These circles represent the mother and father for this particular family. I write their names in the circles and then suggest that since they started this family, they begin by giving me the birthdate and biosociocultural background for each. If one or the other asks who ought to begin, I say, "you decide." As each one says when he or she was born, I write the data under the circle.

Sometime during the eliciting of this chronology, I give another reason why this is useful (other than my becoming familiar with their structure). The fact is that people tend to act in parental roles as they have been acted on. People learn by models rather than from books to a very great extent (Dr. Spock notwithstanding). It is important to know how each present parent was reared and what lessons in child rearing were learned. How the two present parents put together their different backgrounds in child-rearing is easier to understand when the background of each has been described. For instance a German-Jew married to an English-Protestant who live as a nuclear unit produce a very different set of mutual expectations that do two Catholics, for example, Mexican-Americans living in an extended family.

The second item I mention at some point in the chronology is the work of Walter Toman on family constellation. He discovered that one's sibling position greatly influences the kinds of interactions with people one is likely to use in adulthood. For instance, firstborn children are more likely to be leaders rather than followers, while the last ones born are more likely to be followers than leaders. It is no accident that all of the astronauts, except one, were firstborn children. At a family conference conducted by the Philadelphia Child Guidance Clinic, one of the speakers asked the audience to indicate by a show of hands how many were firstborn. Of the roughly 1000 family therapists in that room, about 80 percent were firstborn. That, too, is no accident or random event. It strongly suggests that one's experience in interaction dynamics as a child influences one's adult career.

For each parent, I map out, on the family tree, their sibling position in their family of origin, and then I tell them what Toman would say about their likely adult psychodynamic style with others. I invite them to validate or question the description. Ninety-nine percent of the time the sibling constellation projection is so accurate that it surprises or sometimes even astounds the listener. The secondary gain from this strategy is that it allows you, as the therapist, to point out that doing family therapy is really a science — and not some poorly formulated affair — and that it puts you in the position of having demonstrated your skills.

Besides the data about each parent, which is biosociocultural material (such as religion, ethnic background, social class, values, and general physical health), and the sibling position of each, you need to know about their own parents — whether they are living or dead, still married, separated or divorced, geographically near or distant, and so on. If they are present during this session, of course they can provide the data themselves. I use the space above the two parental circles to record the data about the parents' parents.

Even after having done many, many intakes over the years, I am still impressed by the diversity of family structuring. It is not true that children have two parents, that they live together in a nuclear unit, and that their parents had two parents who lived in nuclear units. The existance of situations that depart from this norm make the norm truly a myth.

You need to know how this particular parental pair met, how they decided to marry, and how they established the division of labor rules within their new unit. Ask whether the children were planned or not, what difference the arrival of each made in the household division of labor, and what the present expectations for each child are. I go about this by asking each child his or her birthdate, what they are expected to do as a family member, and what they have in mind for themselves as adults. I address the questions about age to any child two or above and the question about family expectations to any child four or above. Whether the child answers for himself or herself yields important dynamics about family roles. Also asking about family expectations as opposed to a projected adult career introduces the family to the concept of separateness, connectedness, or solidarity — a concept that so often is the primary issue in family troubles. There is another way to ask this: How much of the time can an individual in this family do his own thing, and how much of the time must he or she contribute total effort toward family goals?

As the children speak for themselves, say who they are and so on, I draw a circle for each, placing the circles in a horizontal line from a stem coming from the parental circles. I use dotted lines to designate half brothers or sisters. You will need to invent your own system to record such information as the number of divorces, adoptions, deaths, and children temporarily living away from the unit in hospitals or schools. The symbols I use work for me, but clinicians need to develop their own systems for recording.

When the chronology is completed, it is time for the therapist to ask what the family sees as the present problem or difficulty. They may or may not come up with the same thing as is listed on the intake or referral form. Don't worry about the discrepancy, if there is one. Another rule to remember is never look at the identified patient, if there is one, when asking what the difficulty is. Look anywhere else — but not at him or her. This reinforces your earlier statements about systems. The remainder of the time will be spent by your clarifying the difficulty. System principles supply you with the analytical framework in which you ask questions to clarify. The overall guiding question is who has the right to do what to whom under what conditions? Violations of the family's norms and expectations produce the signals and symptoms that, in the past, we have called mental illness. Now that sounds terribly simple. It is. The hard part is ferreting out the answers to this question from the complexities of verbal and nonverbal signals and clues that families produce. Another way is to visualize the family's system rules (their rules for each of the role players) as a clear-as-a-bell tone that is possible to hear under conditions of honest, straightforward communication. What troubled families produce, instead, is a whole lot of noise, static, and cacophony that hurts their own eardrums and quite possibly those of their surrounding systems. The therapeutic role, in this analogy, is to produce clear tones and eliminate the noise and static. Insofar as this is achieved, the family can then move forward to making decisions about changes in their interactions and expectations for each of the members.

Part I

CHANGING THE THERAPIST

1.

Bias of Therapists in Family Therapy

Grayce Sills

This selection presents a conceptual framework for viewing bias as an influence emanating from the therapist that alters system behavior in the course of family therapy. A brief review is made of the work done on bias in the areas of experimental research, survey research, and interviewing. Sources and types of bias are discussed and illustrated with clinical instances from family therapy data. Furthermore, it is shown how the injection of bias into family therapy sessions unwittingly alters or fails to alter system behavior. This is followed by a brief discussion of possible strategies for the prevention and control of unfavorable bias.

BIAS AS COMMUNICATIVE BEHAVIOR

In research terms, bias is viewed as a source of error. Hence, bias is to be avoided in every possible way. In interviewing, and in therapy, bias has long been recognized as a major factor influencing the present behavior of the interactional pair. In therapeutic work, Sullivan called attention to the significance of the therapist's participation in therapy sessions and made explicit reference to the extraneous injection of unwanted biases.[1] Also, Sullivan called attention to what use could be made of favorable bias. To read any of Sullivan is to become rapidly aware of his own very favorable bias with regard to the dilemmas of human existence.

The essence of bias is that it exists in somewhat unprecise quantities

[1] Harry S. Sullivan, *The Psychiatric Interview,* New York, W. W. Norton Co., 1954, passim.

13

and somewhat vague qualities in and of the actor. In this selection the focus will be on bias as qualitative and quantitative phenomena generated in interaction with the therapist viewed as the protagonist. Furthermore, the scope will be narrowed to include those biases that can be seen to produce negative effects in relation to desired effects. Such a limitation is not meant to imply that bias may not operate favorably in relation to desired effects, but rather to make the same point Hyman does.

Hyman says:

Let it be noted that the demonstration of error marks the advanced state of a science. All scientific inquiry is subject to error, and it is far better to be aware of this, to study the sources in an attempt to reduce it, than to be ignorant of the errors concealed in the data. [2]

EXPERIMENTAL RESEARCH

Rosenthal provides a comprehensive and systematic treatment of experimenter effects in behavioral research. The definition used by him that parallels what in this selection is called bias is:

When the experimenter interacts with the subject his own more enduring attributes, his attitudes and his expectancies, may prove to be significant determinants of the subject behavior. [3]

Rosenthal presents research evidence that "unintended social influence" is related to biosocial, psychosocial, and social psychological attributes of the experimenter. Furthermore, he shows that "unintentional influence" is related to situational factors, structural variables, and certain behavioral variables. In this latter category is included professional status, interpersonal style, kinesic communication, and paralinguistic communication. Another category that demonstrated marked effect on subject response was experimenter expectancy. Merton's familiar concept of the "self-fulfilling prophecy" characterizes this category. Rosenthal provides empirical data to support the hypothesis that expectancy on the part of the experimenter or teacher can influence subject response. Rosenthal further suggests:

If experimenters can, and if teachers can, then probably healers, spouses and other "ordinary people" also can affect the behavior of those with whom they interact by virtue of their expectations of what that behavior will be. [4]

[2]H. H. Hyman, et al., *Interviewing In Social Research,* Chicago, University of Chicago Press, 1954, p. 4.
[3]Robert Rosenthal, *Experimental Effects In Behavioral Research,* New York, Appleton-Century-Crofts, 1967, p. viii.
[4]Ibid, p. 412.

SURVEY RESEARCH

In survey research the question of interviewer bias is a central issue and concern. Most often the problem of bias is conceptualized as observer selectivity. Since survey research does not often involve communications, sometimes the focus for the concern is more narrow. Richardson and Dohrenwend treat the issue this way:

Although trained observers separate observation from interpretation their biases and feelings may well cause them to observe selectively.[5]

These authors posit a combination of expectations and premises that will produce unanticipated responses, hence spontaneity in the subject's response to questions. They suggest that if the interviewer has an informed strong expectation coupled with an informed premise, the more valid the unanticipated responses will be. In their book they develop a useful paradigm of combinations of expectations and premises.[6]

INTERVIEWING AND THERAPY

The interviewing and therapy literature nearly always includes some reference to the issue of bias. Kahn and Cannell define bias as: "The intrusion of *unwanted* or *unplanned* interviewer influence in the interview process.[7]" These authors suggest that the major sources of bias are background characteristics, psychological attributes, and behavior in the interview itself. They present a model of bias in the interview in which the key linking factor is perception. In terms of their three factors given above, they suggest that "behavior in the interview" is most amenable to correction through training.

Watzlawick affirms that variations in the patient's condition may be a partial result of observer bias.

However once it is accepted from a communicational point of view a piece of behavior can only be studied in the context in which it occurs. The terms "sanity" and insanity practically lose their meanings as attributes of individuals. Similarly does the whole notion of "abnormality" become questionable. For now it is generally agreed that the patient's condition is not static but varies with the interpersonal situation as well as with the bias of the observer.[8]

[5]Stephen Richardson and Barbara Dohrenwend, *Interviewing in Social Research,* New York, Basic Books, 1966, p. 14.

[6]Ibid, p. 178.

[7]Robert Kahn and Charles Cannell, *The Dynamics of Interviewing,* New York, Wiley, 1957, p. 59.

[8]Paul Watzlawick, J. H. Beavin, and Don Jackson, *Pragmatics of Human Communication,* New York, W. W. Norton, 1967, pp. 46–47.

Lederer and Jackson, in discussing marriage therapy, suggest pitfalls to be avoided, such as forcing ones own values on the clients, siding with one of the marital partners, playing a judicial role, and making hurried assumptions about strengths or weaknesses in the clients.[9]

Haley states that: "Therapists of all schools particularly emphasize being fair and not taking sides with any one family member."[10]

Therefore, bias is seen in the behavioral sciences as unwitting, unintentional intrusion into the behavioral matrix of some attribute, characteristic, or behavior that evokes an unplanned response.

A CONCEPTUAL FRAMEWORK
FOR BIAS IN FAMILY THERAPY

Bias occurs when there is unwitting or unintentional and unwanted social influence introduced into the family therapy session by the therapist. Such a definition rules out what are commonly referred to as "theoretical biases," for such biases operate for a greater extent wittingly and knowingly. Furthermore, the major emphasis will be on biases that are unwanted and produce undesired consequences. It is noted here that there may be biases operating unwittingly and unintentionally that produce favorable or desired effects. This category will not be dealt with here.

Conceptually, therapeutic work with families is interaction on a different level from what typically occurs in the usual one-to-one relationship or even that of dyads in treatment together with one therapist. The fast-moving pace of families often involves interaction among three or more persons. Therefore, the complexity of the interaction makes the intrusion of biasing phenomena in one respect less important, that is, it is possible for the family to ignore the intrusion and go merrily on its way. In another respect when systems theory is used as a theoretic base for therapy, the unwanted intrusion can disturb the systems patterns of operation, hence the situation is markedly different as a consequence of the disrupting input.

THE CONCEPTUAL FRAMEWORK

First, it is stated that the family operates as a system. Parents, children, and other family members are subsystems that comprise this total system.

[9]William Lederer and Don D. Jackson, *Mirages of Marriage,* New York, W. W. Norton, 1967, pp. 405–439.
[10]Jay Haley, *Strategies of Psychotherapy,* New York, Grune & Stratton, 1963, p. 170.

When there have been signals of system disruption, the family therapist is called in to diagnose the trouble and strategize for change. The hypothesis here is that the therapeutic work is best accomplished if the system works out its own changes, shifts in behavior, and operating modes. Therefore, the framework implies a therapist committed to systems theory as a base for the work. Further implicated in this statement is that inputs from the therapist that perpetuate the systems' disruption or sidetrack the systems' struggle for reequilibrating modes can be biasing. Thus, the framework is stated as follows.

1. There is a family system in some state of disruption.

2. The family therapist is called on to facilitate reequilibration.

3. Inputs emanate from the therapist in the system that are unwitting, unplanned, and unwanted in view of the goals of therapy.

4. The system responds by being sidetracked, refusing to work, perpetuating problematic patterns, and so forth.

SOURCES AND TYPES OF BIAS IN FAMILY THERAPY

This article does not purport to explicate all the sources and types of bias in family therapy. Thus, the focus will be limited to those that come into view as a part of a workshop experience with family therapy.[11]

The sources of bias in family therapy are linked to the same attributes, characteristics, and behavior as have already been discussed from the existing literature. The types of bias seem somewhat different in family therapy as opposed to other kinds of therapy or other types of behavioral interaction.

Based on the clinical data the following categories have been derived.

1. Coalition biases.

2. Dynamics biases.

3. Social biases.

COALITION BIASES

Haley suggests that a most immediate question when the therapist enters the power struggle in a family is: Where will he fit into coalition

[11]Credit goes to those faculty and members of the workshop who generously shared their errors with the writer. They were Sue Kennedy, Shirley Smoyak, Ruth Roberts, Cosma Rhinehart, Leitha Liberman, and Janet Jackson. The writer's own errors also are shared in the clinical instances.

patterns? He states that the therapist needs to not let himself be provoked into coalitions with family members that are instigated by symptoms or family distress.[12]

Coalition can be seen as arising from at least three sources: age, sex, and as "pull for the underdog" bias. Clinical examples are shared to illustrate each of the foregoing.

> *Age.* A family therapist describes a family discussion with natural grandmother, mother, and children present. The focus is on the "Hippies" and teen age rebellion. The therapist is age-matched with the mother, and finds that she is agreeing with mother's views. In the tape recording of this interview, and in the observer notes, both verbally and nonverbally indicated the coalition with the mother.

The system behavior was momentarily changed as the other family members perceived the coalition. The problematic piece of this instance of bias is that it offers the members of the family a view of the therapist that is unwanted in terms of the goals of therapy.

> *Sex.* The sex of the therapist may operate in an unwitting way to promote same-sex coalitions. The following conversation is from a family therapy session where the therapist is female.

Mother: I want the family life to be more tolerable.

Therapist: Be more specific; what would be more tolerable?

Mother: I don't understand. Just more bearable I guess.

Therapist: Give me a specific behavior that would make things more tolerable.

Mother: I don't understand.

Therapist: For instance, if you have on a tight girdle and you take it off, that's a specific behavior that makes a given situation more tolerable.

Mother (laughs and says): Now I know what you mean.

Here the therapist unwittingly aligned herself with the mother on the basis of an example that only women could understand. The husband and other family members were then excluded by the "femaleness" of the example. This was particularly unfortunate in this family for the father, who was in an almost-stable "one down" position with regard to his wife. The tape recordings of this session show that the father did not participate in the discussion for the next 35 minutes. The "unintended influence" had closed him out.

[12]Op. cit. pp. 170–171.

"Pull for the underdog"

Particularly in familes where there is a member identified as patient, there is often engendered in the therapist a tendency to see that person as a victim. Such a perception can lead to what has been labeled "the rescue fantasy" in individual psychotherapy. In family therapy it often leads to advocacy for the identified patient on the part of the therapist. Such a stance is illustrated in the following example.

> The J. family is composed of father, mother, and three children, ages 18, 14, and 10. Mr. J has a long history of irresponsible acts, borrowing large sums of money, and the like. At the present time he is designated as legally incompetent. Mrs. J. reminds him, the family, and the therapist of this fact very often. The therapist decides that Mr. J. needs assistance and proceeds to become his advocate as the following exchange demonstrates.

Wife: I only have two choices when he goes out and borrows. I got to pay it, or I cannot pay it.

Therapist: Are there other possibilities?

Wife: None

Husband: If I didn't do it to start with.

Therapist: Suppose you make a deal. If he does borrow or hock things, he has to work to pay for it.

Husband: OK.

Wife: Tell me more.

The interchange that followed the above piece lasted for about 20 minutes. During this time the therapist and the wife tried to bargain *about* the husband's behavior. The husband did not participate. The therapist playing the advocacy role for the husband served only to increase his felt "incompetence." Hence, what began as a benign maneuver, because of the bias inherent in it, succeeded only in perpetuating ongoing patterns in family system.

Another instance is cited. The D. family is composed of a husband, wife, and three children: two girls and one boy. Mrs. D. was the identified patient and used symptoms as in an effort to control the behavior of other family members. The husband was viewed by the therapist as quite competent but usually being "put down" by the amorphous communication of his wife. In the discussion that follows, Mr. D. is telling Mrs. D. that he will do what she wants, that is, go back to school, get a secondary degree for teaching credentials, work in the summers for an M. A. in a field of his choice, but continue to live in her hometown (her wishes).

Mrs. D.: Let's just cancel the whole mess!

Therapist: He didn't say that!

As heard on the tape recording, the therapist's voice was raised and sharp. Clearly the bias for the perceived "underdog" was operating. Furthermore, in these data it was noted that the therapist was frequently reinforcing the husband and asking the wife for further classification in rather brisk preemptory tones. Again, playing advocate for any member of the family system, when done unwittingly and unintended, only provides for combination of patterns that have already demonstrated their lack of usefulness.

Still another instance is cited. The therapist was working with a family in which a complementary pattern of integration was operating with the wife "one up" and the husband "one down." The exchange follows:

Husband: What do you really want from me?

Wife: To live through — to be all the things I never could.

Husband: You wanted to live through me?

Wife: I also expected some return, gratitude, affection consideration, loving.

Therapist: So you expected him to be affectionate and love you *and yet* during your pregnancy you said that when you got home from work you felt miserable so you turned out the lights and went to bed.

In this instance the therapist's use of "so" and "yet" the bias in favor of the husband is expressed. The therapist participates in the role of advocate of the husband. Such participation, when minimal and shifting, is likely not disruptive to the system. However, in this instance, it was after listening to the tape and hearing the voice that recognition of bias occurred.

DYNAMIC BIASES

Dynamic biases refer to several ideas. First, those the therapist develops at an intuitive level are operated on *as if* the ideas had been confirmed in fact. The second includes those ideas that stem from a therapeutic orientation different from the one the therapist is currently attempting to utilize. The first category can be illustrated by the following exchange between a therapist and supervising therapist.

The family the therapist was working with had a marital dyad where the wife did most of the "one-upping." During the supervision of the third family session, the supervisor asked the therapist, "How did Mr. Elizabeth respond to that?" Elizabeth was the wife's name.

In the above, the "Freudian slip" is seen as a cue to the supervisor's unwitting unintended bias. Had the slip not occurred, been noticed, and accounted for, the quality of the supervision would have suffered. An illustration of the second type of dynamic bias where the therapist is attempting to learn a therapeutic orientation, different from one previously learned, is demonstrated in the following example.

The family is large with nine family members. The identified patient is a 16-year-old daughter. The therapist is speaking: "Actions affect the entire family. Three of you identified the *problem* as Minnie's taking things."

In the above illustration it can be seen that although the therapist was attempting to use a system approach, in fact, the family was reinforced in their "problem" orientation. Hence, the earlier theoretic basis intruded, unintended, to support the family's bias that they only had *one* problem — the identified patient.

Another illustration can be made of the bias emanating from shifting orientations. The therapist in this instance was a nurse with a background in public health. Her "modus operandi" was to get families to make decisions about health problems and take responsibility for their actions. In the family session, the husband and wife were focusing on the issue of the husband's smoking. The therapist immediately tried to get the dyad to "solve the problem."

The bias here operated to prevent the therapist from seeing that "meta rules" have to first be established before any negotiation on agreement or bargain could take place. Hence, in response to the therapist's bias, the dyad did not succeed at a task, and the pattern of nonagreement is reinforced.

SOCIAL BIASES

This category refers to those biases that stem from the social positions and social roles that the therapist occupies in addition to his professional role.

The above can be illustrated by a therapist who, in attempting intervention in a family with a young adolescent boy, says, "I wouldn't tolerate that from my son!" The referrent is the boy's behavior toward his mother, which is loud, noisy, and somewhat disrespectful.

Clearly, the issue above is *not* the moral rectitude of the son's behavior but, instead, the sequential pattern of behavior within the family system that accommodates such behavior. The therapist's social role as "father of a son" leads him to express his "fatherly bias" toward the son in a family not his own. Not only does such bias interfere with seeing the system operate and facilitating the system's requilibration, but also it comes close to imposing one's value system and style of family life on a family not one's own.

STRATEGIES FOR PREVENTION OF BIAS

Two major types of bias seem to stand out in family therapy: the coalition biases and the shift in orientation biases. Both are amenable to correction through careful supervision and through orientation. Through these two methods the development of what Sullivan has so felicitously named the "critical auditor" can take place. Then one is able to provide relatively bias free interaction in therapy.

Novice therapists could be exposed to a variety of error-ridden performances through videotape in an effort to demonstrate the consequences of bias. Adorno's F scale and the Rakeach "open-close minded" scale might facilitate the identification of therapists who have greater potential for error due to bias.

Gunner Myrdal has called attention to "value premises" as factors that operate in all behavioral science efforts. He suggests that explicitly naming the orientational base of values from which one is working is essential to the understanding of any inquiry.[13] Perhaps, Myrdal's concept is useful to family therapists. Novice therapists could be asked to explicate the value premises they hold about families and what family life should be like.

The strategy implicated by definition is that of awareness. Once the bias becomes known it can be edited out of the behavioral repertoire of the therapist.

[13]Gunnar Myrdal, *Asian Drama,* New York, Pantheon Press, 1968, Appendix II, Volume III.

SUMMARY

This selection has presented an interview of the problem of bias in the behavioral sciences and focused specifically on biases that operate with family therapists. Clinical data were used to illustrate instances of bias. Some consequences for the family as a system were pointed out. Strategies for prevention and elimination of bias were suggested.

BIBLIOGRAPHY

Haley, Jay. *Strategies of Psychotherapy,* New York, Grune and Stratton Co., 1963.

Hymann, Herbert et al. *Interviewing in Social Research,* Chicago, University of Chicago Press, 1957.

Kahn, Robert and Charles Cannell. *The Dynamics of Interviewing: Theory, Techniques and Cases,* New York, Wiley, 1957.

Lederer, William, and Don Jackson. *Mirages of Marriage,* New York, W. W. Norton Co., 1968.

Myrdal, Gunnar. *Asian Drama,* New York, Pantheon Press, 1968.

Richardson, Stephen and Barbara Dohrenwend. *Interviewing in Social Research,* New York, Basic Books, 1966.

Rosenthal, Robert. *Experimenter Effects in Behavioral Research,* New York, Appleton-Century-Crofts, 1957.

Sullivan, Harry S. *The Psychiatric Interview,* New York, W. W. Norton Co., 1954.

Watzlawick, P., J. H. Beavin, and Don D. Jackson. *Pragmatic of Human Communication,* New York, W. W. Norton Co., 1967.

2.

The Use of Analogies in Introducing the Systems Concept to Families in Therapy

Imelda Wiltz Clements and Diane Buchanan

During the past decade the systems concept has revolutionized both the physical and psychosocial sciences. This has been accomplished in psychology by modifying the traditional intrapsychic orientation that had focused attention in intrapsychic variables, often at the expense of social, psychological, and situational components. The systems concept went further than the intrapsychic theory and helped explain the mysterious behavior that resulted when two or more persons related to one another. In order to show how systems theory can be introduced into family therapy sessions, a brief discussion of systems theory, human systems in particular, and characteristics of systems will be discussed. Examples of family systems analogies designed to assist the nurse-family therapist in presenting the systems concept to low-articulate families will be outlined followed by an analysis of each.

SYSTEMS CONCEPT

A system is a complex of components in mutual interaction or as a set of units containing common properties that are conditioned by or dependent on the state of the other units ([1]Bertalanffy, p. 708, Miller, p. 200). One example of this is the family as a system and the individual family members as the units that are related to one another.

In discussing this concept it is important to realize that a system may itself be a subsystem or unit of a larger system, and that it similarly may very well have subsystems within it. A system may also be related to a number of systems. An example is nuclear family B, which is a subsystem of the extended family A, and also a subsystem of the larger community in which they live. The term "related to" indicates that there is opportunity for an exchange between the systems and that this is what an open system is, that is, a system in which there is an opportunity for an exchange of matter-energy or information with the environment. Living systems such as human-social systems are examples of open systems. When there is an opportunity for exchange of matter-energy in an open system, the open system is able to take in or import energy from its outside environment, to utilize some of this energy within its system, and to give out or export energy back into the outside environment. It is through this exchange of energy that a system is able to introduce and take part in change both inside and outside its system. This latter point — that change can occur inside as well as outside the system — leads one to consider how knowledge about systems and systems theory can be utilized by a therapist and the family in therapy in bringing about change in and out of the family system.

THE NURSE THERAPIST AND SYSTEMS ANALOGIES

In addition to seeing herself as the resource person and official observer in therapy sessions, the nurse-family therapist must be a model of clear communication. It also is important that she teach the family how to achieve clear communication themselves. She must be sure in her own mind what she wants to communicate to the family in the teaching process and also to state this in terms that will be clear and acceptable to the family. The therapist must construct and interpret the action of therapy in order to introduce the family to new techniques in communication. Various cultures, ages, educational, and intellectual levels are met in family therapy. Each family requires different amounts of adaptation on the part of the therapist in order to convey the systems concept to them. The highly articulate family may readily grasp the concept, whereas the lower articulate families will often find the concept confusing and difficult to understand. An analogy may be used to convey effectively the systems concept to these families.

CRITERIA FOR SYSTEMS ANALOGY

In developing an analogy to convey the systems concept to the low-articulate family, all relevant characteristics of living systems should be contained in the analogy.

Briefly these are the following:

1. A living system is composed of units or parts. These parts are related to one another and contribute to the total system. Change in one part results in change in other parts, thus affecting the whole system.

2. A living system is open, allowing an exchange of matter-energy to occur with its environment. It permits input and output to pass through its boundaries and throughput to occur within its boundaries. This cycle of events must be continuous for the system to exist.

a. Input into a system contains information, which may be positive and/or negative feedback, as well as energy. The information is a signal to the system about its environment and about its own functioning as related to its environment. The system can accept or reject the incoming information or energy. This act is called coding.

b. Throughput is accomplished by the system accepting and utilizing the incoming energy and information for output and also for storing an adequate amount to draw on to restore its own energy and repair any breakdowns within the system, thus preventing chaos and/or death (entrophy) to the system.

c. Output from the system is also in the form of information and energy.

d. The input and output of energy from and to the environment must remain at a ratio that stays about the same, thus maintaining a steady state for the system.

3. As a living system grows, the parts within the system develop and evolve to greater specialization of function (differentiation). It is through this evolution that the system achieves its steady state.

4. A living system can reach its final goal or state from varying initial conditions and by many different paths (equifinality).

ANALYSIS OF ANALOGIES USING SYSTEMS CRITERIA

The following analogies were developed by members in the Family Workshop for Advanced Psychiatric Skills and were generously shared for the purpose of this selection. The analogy will be presented first, followed by a short critique.

ANALOGY NO. 1

The family is a system much like an orchestra playing Brahm's Lullaby. All the members of the orchestra work together to produce a beautiful rendition. During the rendition the celloist turns to the wrong page and starts playing a different part of the song than the rest of the orchestra. This makes a very stressful situation for the other members, the rendition flounders, and musical chaos ensues.

The orchestra members may react by trying to play louder and drown out the celloist, or the celloist may stop playing. Another alternation may be that the orchestra members stop, help him find his place, and then continue with the music in unison.

All members begin playing again, producing a beautiful rendition of Brahm's Lullaby to the enjoyment of the audience.[1]

Analysis of analogy no. 1

1. System composed of parts —
The conductor and members make up the parts of the system — the orchestra. Change in the system was demonstrated by the celloist turning the wrong page and playing a different part of the song. Stress was produced in the other members thus affecting the whole system with musical chaos.

2. Open system —
a. Input — feedback in the form of stimulation received from the audience; practice, knowledge, and abilities brought in by individual members; and coding — accepting and rejecting the feedback, knowledge, and energy.
b. Throughput — the blending together of all the input, then stopping and finding the place in the sheet of music, drawing from storage any extra needed information, storing extra input, and then blending the needed input and what was drawn from storage into a beautiful rendition.
c. Output — beautiful rendition of Brahm's Lullaby.
d. Steady ratio — correction of celloist's mistake allowed ratio to remain steady.

3. Differentiation — As each member becomes more experienced he is able to cope with and correct a mistake, alone or with other members, thus again achieving a steady state.

4. Equifinality — it was possible to produce a beautiful rendition of Brahm's Lullaby despite added stress on the members during the playing of the piece.

ANALOGY NO. 2

A person executing a golf swing illustrates a system. Change in any one of the identified parts — head, shoulders, arms, wrists, hands, legs, or

[1]Analogy developed by Imelda W. Clements.

feet — will be felt in each other part and will have an effect on the direction and speed of the ball. If each part is not properly balanced, there will be little control over the ball.

If the head is raised, the shoulders and arms are also raised, and the ball may be topped or missed altogether.

If one tends to slice the ball (hit it off to the right), this can be corrected through the system by putting the right foot an inch or two in front of the left foot, thus reestablishing a workable equilibrium.[2]

Analysis of analogy no. 2

1. System composed of parts —
The members of the body and the golf equipment make up the system, which is the person executing a golf swing. How change in one part affects other parts, and the system is well demonstrated.

2. Open System —
   a. Input — the positive and/or negative feedback from companions and others affecting the player, physical condition of the person and the equipment, attitude and the golfers, and coding — accepting or rejecting incoming information and knowledge.
   b. Throughput — drawing on needed input, stored energy, and knowledge to execute a good swing, and also storing up excess input for future use.
   c. Output — a golf swing.
   d. Steady ratio — a successful golf swing depends on adequate input and output.

3. Differentiation — as the golfer becomes more adept, he is able to correct positioning and whatever else might hinder a successful swing.

4. Equifinality — the final goal of a successful golf swing can be accomplished under various conditions just so the golfer has a workable equilibrium.

ANALOGY NO.3

A family operates like a family of birds. Each person has a function in a family. Each bird has a function. In most species, the female sits on the nest to hatch the eggs, and the male brings her food. After the young are hatched, both parents bring them food. The task of the young is to learn to fly and eventually care for themselves. If the female did not cooperate and hatch the eggs, or if the male refused to bring her food, the system would

---

[2]Analogy developed by JoAnn McKay, one of the participants in the U. of New Mexico Family Therapy Workshop.

suffer. The same is true with human families. The behavior of one member affects everyone in the family. As the parent birds continue to function after the babies leave the nest, so can the human family exist and its system when a member leaves home.[3]

Analysis of analogy no. 3

1. System composed of parts —
The bird family is the system made up of its parts — the individual birds. Change in the system is demonstrated by one or other parent bird not carrying out prescribed tasks. Stress is inferred.

2. Open system —
   a. Input — food brought in by the father and coding — when the birds' hunger is satisfied, they may reject food.
   b. Throughput — food taken in and stored and/or utilized for energy to carry out designated tasks.
   c. Output — carrying out tasks.
   d. Steady ratio — in order to carry out tasks, there must be a steady adequate intake of food to meet energy needs.

3. Differentiation — as baby birds develop, they take on more complex tasks.

4. Equifinality — since the roles in the bird and animal kingdom are biogenetically patterned it is more difficult to apply the criterion of equifinality to this system.

[3]Analogy developed by Sally Harris, one of the participants in the U. of New Mexico Family Therapy Workshop.

SUMMARY

This selection presented examples of family systems analogies that were designed to assist the nurse-family therapist in presenting the systems concept to low-articulate families.

A brief review of the literature was made in the area of systems. Criteria for analyzing the system analogies was extracted from works reviewed in the systems area and applied to each of the examples of family system analogies presented. The analysis of each analogy was by no means exhaustive, but the intent was for the analysis to serve as a guide in developing other analogies.

BIBLIOGRAPHY

Bertalanffy, Ludwig von. "General System Theory and Psychiatry," *American Handbook of Psychiatry, Vol. III,* New York, Basic Books, Inc., 1966.

Miller, James G. "Living Systems: Basic Concepts," *Behavioral Sciences, Vol. 10,* 1965.

Smoyak, Shirley A. "Toward Understanding Nursing Situations: A Transaction Paradigm," *Nursing Research, Vol. 18: 5,* September-October, 1969.

3.

Relevance of Historical Data in Systems Theory Approach to Family Therapy

Nellie M. Rodgers

The question has been raised as to the relevance of historical data to the systems theory approach to family therapy. This selection attempts to supply a partial answer to that question. Clinical data are cited to support the concepts presented.

We may consider the point that the patient may recover from illness without knowing "why" he got sick, just as one may be "healthy" in the first place without knowing why he developed so.*

History has been defined as "a chronological record of event," "a record of patient's medical background," "an interesting past," "that which is not of current concern."[1] Here the focus is on the relevance of historical data and intrapsychic dynamic history to systems theory approaches in therapeutic endeavors with the family rather than on the properties of mind or treatment of the individual.

Individual psychotherapy has stimulated the emergence of a dynamic model of personality organization and subsequent analysis of those characteristics.[2] Therefore, much emphasis has been placed on the historical background of the individual in order to define the unconscious motivation for one's emotional problems. It is believed that a person's behavior is heavily influenced by his personal, dynamic, and family history. Consequently, the therapist traditionally has striven to collect a wealth of information regarding the patient's past behavior in an attempt to understand and, in time, change his life-style through the transference process and subsequent gain of insight. More and more the idea is being

*Alexander, Gralnick. "Family Psychotherapy: General & Specific Considerations," *American Journal Orthopsychiatry,* **32**, 1962, 525.

[1] Morris, ed., *American Heritage Dictionary of the English Language,* Boston, Houghton Mifflin Co., 1969, p. 625.

[2] Ivan Boszormenyi-Nagy and James Framo, eds., *Intensive Family Therapy,* New York, Harper & Row, 1966, p. 33.

advocated that insight bears little or no relationship to change in behavior and, therefore, has little value in the therapeutic setting as such — that is, if a change in behavior is the desired outcome of therapy.

Ackerman offers a summary of how much individual "insight-seeking" has limited the therapeutic process.

The understanding of the individual advanced somewhat out of context, in terms of the need for a parallel knowledge of the processes of social interaction. Social workers and psychiatrists seemed often to lose contact with social reality; they lacked clarity in distinguishing the real and unreal. They misapplied or used all too loosely such concepts as transference and resistance. There was rushing concentration on the emotional life of the individual, to the extent that the social frame, within which the individual's reactions were to be judged, was lost sight of.[3]

Because of these factors the therapist who has been trained in the procedures of individual psychotherapy may have considerable difficulty in differentiating between significant and inconsequential background data when involved in system theory approaches to family therapy.

FAMILY SYSTEMS CONCEPT

The relationship of the individual to the family is shown in order to enhance the family systems concept. Systems theory incorporates the idea that the total system is more than the sum of its parts. Each part exists in relation to all other parts. Furthermore, disorder has to do with disarrangement, interruption, or some other alteration of these collective parts. When the family is defined as a system, the disequilibrium has its basis in variation or change in the total system as opposed to a "cause-effect" focus on a so-called illness of an individual who functions within that particular family system.

Haley states,

What is evident is the fact that the description of the "individual" is going to change when his relationships are included in the description. If the individual descriptions offered in the past are used the family context must be ignored. What a person does, why he does it, and how he can be changed will appear different if the description shifts from only him in the context in which he is functioning.[4]

Systems theory disallows the individual as a focal point in family therapy. The person identified as the patient is not an isolate but an integral part of a family unit. More specifically, the ills of the individual

[3]Nathan W. Ackerman, "Interpersonal Disturbances in the Family," *Psychiatry, 17,* Nov. 1954, p. 360.
[4]Jay Haley, *Strategies of Psychotherapy*, New York, Grune and Stratton, 1963, p. 152.

are not separable from the ills of the social context he creates and inhabits. Therefore, the therapist cannot pull the individual out of his cultural milieu and label him sick or well.[5] (Concomitant psychotherapy of several family members is also considered as individual in approach by many theoreticians and practitioners.)

Haley believes that family pathology is a result of a power struggle between persons rather than between internal forces.[6] This is consistent with systems theory, which postulates that the relationships between and among family members are multiple, complex, highly mobile, and virtually inseparable. Ferreira states that the individual and the family are inseparable: "Both points of view must be kept together since each represents what the Chinese call a *chien:* a fabled bird with one eye and one wing. Two such birds must unite for flight to be achieved."[7]

INDIVIDUAL VERSUS FAMILY THERAPY

An individual is *not* static. One's patterns of behavior and family relationships are not static. One cannot, therefore, be evaluated and treated without consideration of that person's value and participation as an integral part of the family system.

The preceding comments are in opposition to treatment approaches advocating probing of the unconscious or dealing with transference phenomenon. Instead, the requirement is one of examination of current behavioral and interactional patterns within the family that bear relevance to the existing disruptive forces within the system. Inherent is the delineation and interpretation of expectations of family members relative to role congruence for promotion of harmony in relationships and subsequent systems balance.

Prior interpersonal and intrapsychially based modalities of treatment will not suffice for family therapy. Ackerman reiterates this in the following statement.

If we aspire to the goal of reducing to scientific terms the therapeutic approach to disturbances in family relations, it is necessary to adopt a critical, discriminatory attitude toward changing psychotherapeutic fashions, to avoid stereotyping, treatment methods, and to carefully test out what is specific and non-specific, central or peripheral in these procedures.[8]

[5]*Ibid.* p. 2.
[6]Haley, *Op. cit.,* p. 156.
[7]Antonio Ferreira, "Family Myth and Homeostasis," *Archives of General Psychiatry,* **9,** Nov. 1963, p. 61.
[8]Ackerman, *op. cit.,* p. 360.

Caution is in order lest the writer give inference from the above comments that individual psychotherapy is a vital part of systems therapy approaches in family therapy. Concern in the latter is not *"who* the trouble is" but instead *"what* the trouble is." The individual often cited as the identified patient becomes only the signaler of conflict or stress within the system. The therapist is a consultant to the system assisting the family in identifying and promoting mental health potentials.

CURRENT DATA IS OF THE ESSENCE

According to Peplau,[9] the emphasis in family therapy based on systems theory must be on the unnoticed but *observable* instead of the unnoticed but *inferable*. The therapist must understand the system, be knowledgeable of the established network, eke out strategies for maintaining the interactions and integrations of the unit, establish habits, patterns, and styles of interaction based on *live* data, determine what restricts and promotes growth, and make an attempt to alter, enhance, or modify the network.

When one considers that a sociological perspective suggests that human behavior is shaped, in part, by situations and timing of events, the study of *current* behavioral experiences within the family system becomes imperative in therapeutic endeavors. Analysis of the interface of family behavior patterns, in essence, becomes the pivotal point for therapeutic interventions.

The eminence of current behavioral patterns and complexity of relationships within the family involved in family therapy necessitates the collection of relevant and contemporary data. Delving into historical and/or intrapsychic data with either the identified patient (if designated) or other family members is not only cumbersome but absolutely superfluous if, for no other reason, than the fact that history tends to repeat itself. More exciting is the supposition that working with live material might be more invigorating to the therapy process.

It is preferable to initiate the process (of therapy) in a fresh, unprejudiced way, without historical data obtained separately and at different times. As the group wrestles with its immediate distress, a live type of history emerges that is apt to be more relevant and accurate. . . . As the members become engaged in the therapeutic struggle, selected fragments of background are tossed out and subjected promptly to a process of consensual validation among the family members. . . . The live, pungent, and dramatic quality of spontaneous historical disclosures is a convincing experience. After all, history, in the best sense, is contemporary. Its importance and relevance hinge on its being a vital part of the here and

---

[9]*Notes.* Lecture delivered by Dr. Grayce Sills referring to Hildeperd E. Peplau.

now. Factors of pathogenic influence that have come up out of the past can be traced in the contemporary emotional events of the family. This is the 'live past,' not the 'dead past,' of family life.[10]

The therapist could easily become buried in the history-taking process to the point of losing perspective of the current difficulties of the family or, because the ear is tuned to historical data, not hearing or locating the existing current disequilibrium within the family. Moreover, the potential exists for falling into the snare of focusing on the "disease process" of the "patient" instead of considering the alternatives of behavior within the immediate system or becoming lost in uncovering the etiology of a "mental illness" as opposed to aiding the family in evaluating need for and eking out change.

Historical and intrapsychic information is of little value or significance to the systems theory therapist. Such a therapist recognizes that past behavior carries a connotation of "so what." The past is past. The individual or family in question is involved in *present* relationships, and in a particular and specific situation. Yesterday cannot be recalled or re-lived.

Moreover, securing individual and/or family history prior to the initial family interview may prove to be a detriment to the therapeutic process. Such knowledge may precipitate fusing and negativity or otherwise alter the therapeutic process because of bias or preconceived notions. For example, a novice therapist was hesitant in "pressuring the identified patient for participation" because of prior knowlege of the individual's attempted suicide. Specifically, it was noted that the therapist's fears, related anxiety, and potential guilt modified the approach. More important than the threat of a suicidal attempt (later questioned as a valid supposition) would have been attentive nonevaluative listening for the context of the family's communication.

Naturally, some historical data will be revealed in the process of the therapy sessions. It is unavoidable. At times, utilization of such data will be relevant and valuable to the therapeutic process. An attempt has been made to delineate those instances when historical data should be obtained and employed in systems theory-oriented therapy.

CLINICAL EXAMPLES OF UTILIZATION OF HISTORICAL DATA

There are several instances in which historical data may have relevance and pertinency to family therapy. Clinical data are cited for clarification. 1. Selection of analogy for presentation of systems theory to family. Since this overture is generally made during the first session it is appropriate to have awareness of the family constellation and significant history

[10]N. W. Ackerman, *Treating the Troubled Family,* New York, Basic Books, Inc., 1966, p. 93.

in advance of the visit. A therapist had received a referral of a family of an identified patient on an in-service unit. Conversations with the unit staff revealed that Mrs. R. was extremely paranoid and maintained an active delusional system focused in the areas of radio systems, wiretapping, electric brain waves, and the like. Additionally, Mrs. R. exorbitantly feared electroshock treatments; so much so that other treatment approaches were inhibited. In this instance the selection of electronic devices for an analogic parallel would have been inadvisable.

2. Delineation of serial order of events. In order to facilitate the family's learning that anyone may change or alter an event at any point in the transaction, the therapist must first assist the family in portraying and organizing the details of the event. Mr. K. felt despondent and frightened at times because Mrs. K. displayed anger in the early morning. Both the therapist and Mr. K. were confused as to the exact progression of Mrs. K's. activities on arising and while preparing breakfast. Once the specific sequential order was established during the session Mr. K. noted two points at which an alteration of behavior could be made to decrease the potential of having Mrs. K. "fuss" so early in the morning.

3. Review of historical data to verify or disavow an existing pattern of behavior. The therapist may need to ascertain whether a family member has had experience in a particular area of functioning. In the M. family, T. was a "new" adult family member arriving after a recent discharge from the Army. Both Mr. M (stepfather) and Mrs. M. (mother) were having difficulty adjusting the household routine and schedules to the newcomer in the family. The therapist attempted to ascertain whether Mr. M. had had a prior marriage and/or children in order to determine the need for teaching responsibilities, techniques, and functions of fathering. Discovery of the fact that this was Mr. M.'s first marriage would have indicated the need for such teaching as a part of the therapeutic process. Had it been established that Mr. M. had previously been a father and, therefore, had patterns of fathering established in his repertoire, a different direction of therapy would have ensued.

4. Establishing expectations of the family members. Long-practiced patterns of behavior at times may influence how one views current situations. The parents of G. (a three-year-old identified patient) expressed concern about G.'s "hyperactive" behavior and had given labels such as "schizophrenic," "overaggressive," and the like to that behavior. To the therapist, the child appeared no more active than the average three-year-old. A look into the parents' background revealed that both the father and mother had, as children, experienced very low-key energy expenditure in activity patterns. Both had a very conservative approach to motoristic behavior. For these two the control used in childhood was that of voice

control. The result was that the *normal* behavior for a middle-middle class three-year-old boy was viewed as hyperactive. Indication for direction of therapy was then adjusted accordingly.

5. Comparative or illustrative purposes. The therapist may, at times, wish to have the family look at past behavior to assist in citing possible alternatives of behavior in lieu of what it used to be. Mrs. K. was fearful that Mr. K. would not keep his promise to stay away from his brother-in-law, Mr. B. Mr. K. recalled a similar incident involving another brother-in-law. This was cited as an example of the change that Mr. K. had made in the past. The therapist then used historical data regarding Mr. B. to role play a potential situation in which Mr. K. would encounter Mr. B. Past change was emphasized to encourage future change.

6. Ascertainment of consistency and value of an existing pattern of behavior. Frequently, the therapist may wish to establish how a previously practiced pattern of behavior is coupled to current routines in the system and the related potential for change in that pattern. Mrs. B. was taught that "spotless" housecleaning was a paramount function of a good housewife. This behavior was inherent in Mrs. B.'s daily routine and in the subsequent upbringing of Mrs. B.'s son (by first marriage). Both the son and the stepson (of the second marriage) were expected to clean the house religiously. The importance of this ingrained pattern of behavior to Mrs. B. created considerable friction within the family system. The therapist had to weigh the potential for change in Mrs. B.'s expectations as well as the potential for change in the children (based on historical data) prior to mapping therapeutic strategies in that area of unit function.

7. Apperception of cultural and ethnic differences between the family and the therapist behavior. The therapist must be perceptive to cultural norms and values that would have bearing on therapeutic endeavors. Mr. E. telephoned to cancel future scheduled home visits of the therapist. On the initial visit there was allusion to the potential of divorce of some marital dyads involved in therapy. The therapist was not sensitive to the ethnic code of a Spanish-American, Catholic, middle-class family that says, "We stay together, regardless of the pain or problem" and, therefore, was not again allowed into the home. The opportunity for therapeutic encounter was lost. A more careful assessment of the cultural norms through historical data collection may have alerted the therapist to the potential loss. The approach could then have been altered.

SUMMARY

As viewed by systems theory practitioners of family therapy, historical data — especially of an intrapsychic nature — has a very small place in the therapeutic process. The thrust of therapy should keep in focus the current order of functioning within the family system and should always be open to new information. Focus on past behavior and individual dynamic history becomes secondary to the process of observation and isolation of live behavioral interactional transactions — the latter encroaching on anticipated change within the family system.

The reported examples of appropriate utilization of historical data are not necessarily exhaustive in category but instead are intended as a citation of the limited scope of such data in dynamic family therapy.

BIBLIOGRAPHY

Ackerman, Nathan W. "Interpersonal Disturbances in the Family," *Psychiatry,* **17,** Nov. 1954, 359-68.

Ackerman, Nathan W., *Treating the Troubled Family,* New York, Basic Books, Inc., 1966.

Boszormenyi-Nagy Ivan, and James Framo, eds. *Intensive Family Therapy,* New York, Harper and Row, 1966.

Ferreira, Antonio. "Family Myth and Homeostasis," *Archives of General Psychiatry:* **9,** Nov. 1963.

Haley, Jay. *Strategies of Psychotherapy,* New York, Grune and Stratton, 1963.

Morris, ed. *American Heritage Dictionary of the English Language,* Boston: Houghton Mifflin Co., 1969.

Peplau, Hildeperd. Lecture notes, Dr. Grayce Sills, July 29, 1971.

4.

The Therapist was a Gringa

Barbara Croddy

This article deals with a problem currently dealt with in family therapy: that of cultural incongruence between family and therapist. Conditions responsible for the increased magnitude of this problem will be postulated. Clinical examples of various aspects of family therapy in which cultural differences were problematic will be presented along with interventions used.

Following the report of the Joint Commission on Mental Illness and Health in 1961 and the subsequent allocation of federal and state monies, comprehensive mental health centers have been established across our nation. This has made psychiatric help available to more people than ever before and, in part, accounts for the increase in the number of persons receiving psychiatric care. Not only has there been a change in the number of persons seeking help with emotional disturbances but, as the stigma of mental illness fades, as the mass media forces the general public into awareness of disturbances within family life, and as members of social agencies and institutions become more adept at recognizing and referring psychiatric problems, a change in the cultural composition of psychiatric clientele has been noted. A study done at Boston State Hospital indicates the present-day occupational level of patients is significantly lower than that of the norm group used in the comparative study.[1] Differences are apparent in areas other than occupational levels. Our country is a cultural matrix of many subcultures. Inherent in this is a predisposition to conflict. Freud drew attention to the use of small subcultures as scapegoats to drain off the hostility of better-structured in-groups. Se-

[1]Anne Parsons, *Belief, Magic, and Anomie Essays in Psychosocial Anthropology*, New York, The Free Press, 1969, p. 132.

ward agrees when she indicates that the greatest threat to the continued health of a simple culture comes from outside contacts.[2] Maintenance of a culture's intactness is necessary for continued adjustment of its members. As rejected minority groups strive to emerge and attain greater status the conflict becomes more apparent. With these ideas and facts in mind the increasing numbers of lower-class persons seeking professional help is not surprising. The dilemma occurs when one realizes that most of the professional help givers in the mental health field have middle-class origins.

Why cultural differences between therapist and client may be problematic will now be explored. A social cure that will result in a more satisfying and productive life in the community is the goal of intensive psychotherapy. For therapy to be successful, the client and the therapist must have between them interlocking cultural patterns.[3] Behavior that deviates from the social norm is labeled sick, crazy, or abnormal by the general citizenry. Without knowledge of the cultural norm it is impossible for the therapist to recognize the deviation. Because middle-class values have served as reference points for the middle-class scientists, distinctive subcultural features, characteristic of lower classes, have been overlooked.[4] It is the responsibility of the therapist to know about his client's social norms and to consider them relevant to the treatment process.[5]

Carl Rogers believes ". . . it is the presence of certain attitudes in the therapist which are communicated to and perceived by his client, that affect success in therapy."[6] These attitudes, which he designates as (1) congruence or genuineness, (2) complete acceptance, and (3) empathetic understanding would be difficult if not impossible to attain if one had no appreciation of the conditions of the client's socialization process.

Midelfort strongly expresses the need for the therapist and the patient to have similar ethnic and religious backgrounds. A pioneer in the area of family therapy, he attributed successful therapy to the fact that the cultural background of the therapist and the patient were the same.[7] A therapist of the same race does offer his patients, according to Seward, the possibility of greater freedom and deeper identification.[8]

---

[2]Georgene Seward, *Psychotherapy and Cultural Conflict*, New York, The Ronald Press Co., 1956. pp. 17–22, 32.

[3]*Ibid.* p. 61.

[4]Seward, *op. cit.*, p. 79.

[5]Parsons, *op. cit.*, p. 323.

[6]Carl R. Rogers, "Client-Centered Therapy" in *American Handbook of Psychiatry*, Silvano Arieti, Ed., New York, Basic Books, Inc., 1966, Vol. III, p. 184.

[7]C. F. Midelfort, *The Family In Psychotherapy*, New York, McGraw-Hill, Inc., 1957, pp. 1–12.

[8]Seward, *op. cit.*, p. 153.

Parsons suggests the importance of bringing intimates of the patient into the therapeutic situation with the purpose that someone from the same culture could interpret significant aspects of the patient's experience.[9] Ackerman lists among the functions of a family therapist certain roles that could never be fulfilled if cultural differences were ignored. These include the role of reality tester, parent figure, clarifier of conflict, and personifier of family health model.[10]

Cultural incongruence, as it affects nurse-patient relationships, is compared to a computer system by Smoyak.[11] She states that the nurse and the patient are programmed by their socializing agents and if the data differs when fed into the computer the results will be "no match." Adjustments will have to be made in the programming if the data are to be acted on and useful outputs produced.

At a workshop in family therapy this writer was faced with the task of reprogramming herself in an effort to effect a meaningful relationship with a Spanish-American family. Clinical examples used to demonstrate the significance of cultural differences between families and therapists have been compiled from data collected during the Advanced Workshop in Psychiatric Nursing Skills.[12] The families referred to in this paper were of Spanish-American descent and the therapists were white Anglo-Saxons.

Although aspects of cultural dissimilarity permeated most of the family sessions, this article deals with the problems presented in four general areas of therapy: goal expectations, establishment of rapport, communication styles, and acceptance of ideas.

GOAL EXPECTATIONS

Among the goals of the family therapist are (1) to observe problem areas in patterned family interactions and (2) to help the family to try new ways.[13] The practical goal of family therapy, according to Boszormenyi-Nagy, is the attainment of more meaningful relationships for the family members. He lists more specific goals as the "removal of symptoms," enabling children to obtain "workable models for identification," the "removal of specific obstacles" that interfere with the

[9]Parsons, *op. cit.,* p. 322.

[10]Nathan Ackerman, "Family Therapy" in *American Handbook of Psychiatry,* Silvano Arieti, Ed., New York, Basic Books Inc., 1966, Vol. III, p. 206.

[11]Shirley A. Smoyak, "Cultural Incongruence, Some Effects on Nurses' Perceptions," *Nursing Forum,* Vol. 7, No. 3 1969. Pp. 234–238.

[12]Credit is gratefully given to those members of the workshop who shared their data with this writer. They were Inelda Clements, Mrs. Shirley Harrington, and Miss Frecia Kelly. Data from the writer's own experience are also included.

[13]Dr. Grayce Sills, lecture notes, Advanced Workshop in Psychiatric Nursing Skills, July 1970.

family relational growth, the "freedom to raise and resolve controversial issues," and "improvement of the family's interchange with the community."[14] These goals were certainly not what the families visited by the nurse-therapists had in mind. For instance, one mother's expectations diverged markedly from the therapist's goal. The identified patient in this family was a nine-year-old boy whose mother "had" to walk him to school each day and remain with him until he stopped crying. When the therapists told the mother they had come in response to her call to the Child Guidance Center, she said, *Look Marky, these ladies come to take you to school.* The tendency to focus on the removal of one person's symptoms as the ultimate goal of the family sessions was demonstrated by another mother.

Therapist: What would you like to happen as a result of these family sessions?

Mother: For Richard to stop his habits.

These two families were never able to see the symptoms of their children as signals of disturbances in the family system. With the goals of the family and the therapist so divergent, little progress toward change was made.

ESTABLISHMENT OF RAPPORT

Establishing a useful quality of rapport is one of the first functions of a family therapist.[15] This proved to be a difficult task for those therapists who were unfamiliar with the mores of the Spanish-Americans. Picture an impeccably groomed, attractive, young blonde therapist entering the slum dwelling of a Spanish-American family and saying in her most polite manner, "Where would you have us sit?" The expression on the face of the mother was one of utter puzzlement. A similar quality of disbelief was apparent in the therapist as she attempted to get a picture of the family constellation that consisted of a mother, an adult daughter and her two preschool children, a teenage daughter, three sons, ages 17, 9, and 3 years a 20-year-old male friend, and an adult male whom the mother introduced as her brother and the children called "Daddy." The climate quickly became one of mutual shock and disbelief, culminating in the mother's hostile imperative to "Just go, we don't understand. Tell them to send someone Spanish." A hurried but intensive study of the life of Mexican families helped the therapist to gain reentrance into the home; however, a working relationship was never full achieved.

---

[14]Ivan Boszormenyi-Nagy & Framo, James (Eds.) *Intensive Family Therapy,* New York, Harper & Row, 1966, pp. 128, 133–134.

[15]Ackerman, *op. cit.*

When the families are of a socially rejected minority, the therapist must be prepared to meet the problems intrinsic to this situation.[16] Another family, during the second visit of the therapist, was having difficulty seeing the relationship between what the nurse was saying and what they saw as the problem. "We decided to quit this. *They* don't want to help Spanish people anyway." Further conservation revealed the therapist had been incorporated into the "they" that was composed of the Cerebral Palsy Foundation, the Arthritis Foundation, the federal food stamp program, and other agencies seen by the family as nonhelping. Hoggart says the very poor see "them" as the world of bosses, policemen, and public officials who are numerous and powerful.[17] Some cultural conflicts arise through the stereotyping learned by both the therapist and the patient. These stereotypes must be examined and reevaluated before solid rapport can be established. The therapist may or may not choose to discuss this.[18] It was necessary, in the case just mentioned, for the nurse-therapist to discuss openly her lack of knowledge concerning the ways of the Spanish-Americans and to place verbally the mother in the "driver's seat." After this no further mention of discontinuing therapy was made.

COMMUNICATION STYLES

The induction of a therapist into a family group requires adjustments on his part to the particular subculture that the family represents. This includes adopting the language style of the family.[19] One nurse had much difficulty conveying the idea of family compromise. The father of the family finally said, "You keep saying negotiate, bargain, those are business terms. What do they have to do with our family life?" When the nurse realized it was her terminology that was the barrier to communication she was able to find words acceptable to the head of the hourse, and thus put her ideas across.

Frequently several rephrasing attempts were necessary before a therapist could express herself in a way that the family understood. The following example illustrates one such time. The nurse wanted the mother to see the connection between two behavioral changes in her son that occurred on the same day.

Mother: Richard started doing those habits again on Tuesday.

Therapist: What clues do you have about it starting on Tuesday?

[16]Seward, *op. cit.*, p. 151.
[17]Richard Hoggart, *The Use of Literacy*, London, 1951, Chapter 3.
[18]Seward, *op. cit.*
[19]Salvador Minuchin, et al., *Families of the Slums: An Exploration of their Structure and Treatment*, New York, Basic Books, Inc., 1967, pp. 285–286.

Mother: I saw him doing it.

Therapist: Why do you think he happened to begin on Tuesday?

Mother: I saw him doing it Tuesday afternoon.

Therapist: I'm not making myself clear. For what reason do you think it began on Tuesday?

Mother: I don't know.

Workshop participants spent much time developing analogies to communicate to the families with whom they were working the idea of the family as a dynamic system in which the behavior of each member affects the behavior of each other member and, therefore, affects the functioning of the family as a whole. These attempts met with limited success among the Spanish-Americans. The only attempt that at least partially communicated the idea was the description of pain in one part of the body causing pain in other parts and discomfort to the total person. Even this analogy required some alteration to eliminate aspects that conflicted with the Mexican superstition concerning rapid heart beating.

ACCEPTANCE OF IDEAS

To be effective the therapist must be sufficiently flexible to assume the cultural perspective of those with whom he is working.[20] Middle-class Americans, for the most part, expect and encourage autonomous behavior from their children. This is not a part of the socialization process for the Spanish-American youngsters as was demonstrated on several occasions.

Therapist: Who makes the decisions in this family?

Mother: I do, my husband and I.

Therapist: Do the children ever have a voice in decision making?

Mother: No. (puzzled and almost angry.)

And at another time:

Therapist: Have you given any thought to when it is alright for him to decide for himself?

Mother: No, I don't want him to have his own way.

It was necessary for the therapist to accept the reality of this situation and work within its boundaries. Eventually, the mother decided that when her son was 21 he could make his own decisions. The nurse then tried to instill

[20]Seward, *op cit.,* p. 260.

the idea that having some practice by making some small decisions during the intervening years might be helpful. There was never any indication that she accepted this idea.

For the Spanish-Americans, attitudes toward being ill and being well are expressed in religious, familial, and economic patterns. These people believe they are in God's hands, which makes them resistant to active conscious attempts to change their way of life.[21] Having this information was helpful to the nurse therapist at the session during which the mother was expressing doubts as to the value of the therapy.

Mother: I guess we'll just quit. Richard has stopped his habits for two days now.

Therapist: What if they begin again in the fall when school starts?

Mother: We'll just take a chance. It's all in God's hands anyway.

Therapist: You are right. Ultimately it is up to God. But the Lord helps those who help themselves.

Mother: Yah.

The fact that the therapist accepted instead of rejected the mother's idea was partly responsible for her decision to go on with the therapy sessions.

The influx of people from various subcultures into family therapy situations requires adaptation on the part of the therapists. Having a therapist of the same ethnic and religious background might be considered ideal; however, this is seldom possible. There may, in fact, be some therapeutic value for the family members of one culture to find themselves accepted by a member of another culture. This often allows the person to better accept himself as a member of the subculture.[22] The experience of working with families of a cultural background different from one's own, vividly highlights the need for consideration of these differences if a therapeutic relationship was to develop.

[21]Julian Samora, "Conceptions of Health and Disease Among Spanish-Americans," *American Catholic Sociological Review*, Winter 1961, **22**, 315.
[22]Seward, *op. cit.*, p. 256.

BIBLIOGRAPHY

Ackerman, Nathan W. "Family Therapy," *American Handbook of Psychiatry*, Silvano Arieti, Ed., New York, Basic Books, Inc., Vol. III, 1966.

Boszormenyi-Nagy, Ivan, and James Framo (Eds.). *Intensive Family Therapy*, New York, Harper & Row, 1966.

Hoggart, Richard. *The Use of Literacy*, London, 1951.

Midelfort, C. F. *The Family In Psychotherapy*, New York, McGraw-Hill, Inc., 1957.

Minuchin, Salvador et al. *Families of the Slums: An Exploration of Their Structure and Treatment*, New York, Basic Books, Inc., 1967.

Parsons, Anne. *Belief, Magic, and Anomie: Essays in Psychosocial Anthropology*, New York, The Free Press, 1969.

Rogers, Carl R. "Client-Centered Therapy," American *Handbook of Psychiatry*, Silvano Arieti, Ed., New York, Basic Books, Inc., 1966.

Samora, Julian. "Conceptions of Health and Disease Among Spanish-Americans," *American Catholic Sociological Review*, Winter, 1961.

Seward, Georgene. *Psychotherapy and Cultural Conflicts*, New York, The Ronald Press Co., 1956.

Smoyak, Shirley A. "Cultural Incongruence, Some Effects on Nurses' Perceptions," *Nursing Forum*, Vol. 7, No. 3, pp. 234–238, 1967.

Sills, Grayce. Lecture notes, Advanced Workshop in Psychiatric Nursing Skills, 1970.

Part II

EXPANDING FRAMES OF REFERENCE

5.

"We Are Our Choices"

Marilyn Garin

"We are our choices." So says Sartre, in his existential frame of reference. People end up being what they choose because they end up living these choices out in their daily lives. Sartre continues by saying; "It is therefore senseless to think of complaining since nothing alien has decided what we feel, what we believe, or what we are."[1]

In coming to clinicians for help people do not "complain" about the choices they have made, instead people seem confused and controlled by their choices; they are not aware of nor in command of their destinies. When the choices are in control, they often become defined as necessities. The various unique methods people have for defining necessity are fascinating. There is movement, however, from fascination to distress when these necessities begin to rule and run people's lives.

This selection presents cases of defined necessity in various family systems and demonstrates how these necessities aid to the dysfunctioning of the system and what routes of intervention the therapist may draw on in these situations. Since people are their choices, they have the prerogative to change. The process of change also will be considered. Necessity is defined in a variety of ways. *Webster's Dictionary* defines it thus: (1) Certain and unavoidable character or quality; inevitableness as of death. (2) A compelling force or principle especially one concerned as inherent in nature or in the constitution of things, specifically, a power that determines human action, fate; as, a world governed by necessity. The doctrine of necessity versus the doctrine of Free Will. (3) That which is logically unavoidable, the principle of universal and uniform causation as contrast to chance."[2]

[1]Jean-Paul Sartre, *The Philosophy of Jean-Paul Sartre*, The Modern Library, New York, Random House, p. 278.
[2]*Webster's New International Dictionary, Revised and Unabridged*, 1950.

This is the objective or mandatory necessity that Allen Wheelis talks of in his article, "How People Change." Wheelis says:
— *like natural law which cannot be disobeyed — is that which cannot be suspended. It is derived from forces, conditions, events which lie beyond the self, not subject to choice, unyielding to will and effort. "I wish I had blue eyes," ". . . wish I could fly." Such wishes are irrelevant, choice is inoperative; the necessity impartially constrains. And since it cannot be put aside there's not much arguing about it. "If you jump you will fall — whether or not you choose to fly." There is consensus we don't dwell on it, we accept.*

Both of these sources define necessity as a condition that one cannot change. One takes care of the necessity or pays the price. What is fascinating is how people apply the constraints of necessity to other areas in which they do have a choice, but choose to label the situation a necessity, and soon come to place all the principles of a necessity to this "arbitrary necessity." These types of "arbitrary necessity" were coined and defined by Wheelis. He described them as follows.

They are derived from forces within the personality but are construed to be outside. The force may be either impulse or prohibition: "I didn't want to drink, but I couldn't help it. That is to say, the impulse to drink does not lie within the I. The I, which is of course the locus of choice, does not want to drink, would choose otherwise, but is overwhelmed by an alien force.[3]

These compelling forces, determined by a power outside of the person, takes the responsibility away from the self. But it also takes the choice away from him. The only freedom he is left with is how he will accept this situation. This greatly reduces the range of choice. About the only thing the one subjected to this fate is allowed to decide is how he will accept his fate. Will he do it gracefully, angrily, martyredly? This puts the person who should be in control of his choices in a very subordinate position, practically making him an afterthought to his own life, instead of the essence of it.

There are schools of thought that flow smoothly into this mainstream of determined thought. Determinism dictates that events are determined by a preceding cause. This leads to a cyclic process, and the basic purpose of the process is to keep the energy of the cycle circulating. The cycle exists for its own sake. In deterministic causality, the cause and effect of a situation are interdependent on one another. If there's no cause, there's no effect. In this theory, "because" means "on account of." Night comes, because the sun sets. Or water becomes ice because the temperature goes below 32 degrees.[4] People have some things determined for them at birth: the color of hair, the color of eyes, their sex.

[3]Allen Wheelis, "How People Change," *Commentary,* May, 1969.
[4]Silvano Arieti. *"The Intrapsychic Self,"* London, Basic Books, Inc., 1967, pp. 141–143.

But modern technology is not letting deterministic causality stand in its way. If your eyes are green, with blue contacts you can change a determined fact. If your hair is brown, with bleach you can change a determined fact. If you are born a man, you can have surgery and change a determined fact. Man is saying more and more what he wants, determining his own destiny and not having it deterministically caused.

In social interactions, with people in general and families in particular, the flavor of deterministic causality is often present, as the following examples demonstrate.

1. The mother of a six-year-old, mildly retarded boy "has" to watch him all the time, "because" if she doesn't he will hurt himself. The entire family "has" to go to the barber shop "because" the boy will scream and carry on if they are not there. The entire family "has" to go on a supervised activity of a youth center with the boy "because" the counselors won't be responsible enough. And the boy plays alone after school "because" the other kids play too rough.

2. The uncle of a 19-year-old day-care patient "has" to regulate the boy's money so that the boy's future security is assured.

3. The parents of a 34-year-old, often-hospitalized man "have" to move into the city where he is hospitalized, while the father commutes to his teaching job, both in summer and in winter, so they can be aware of what is going on with him. They "have" to be so aware that they have moved within sight of the hospital.

4. In a family of four children, the three children under 11 "must" take a two-hour nap every day of the summer vacation to ensure that they are rested up for all the summer activities.[5]

These are examples of necessities in various family systems. The necessities have been defined by the system itself and defined so often and so long that they believe that it has to be so. The necessities seem almost like a cycle. In some of the well-established necessity cycles, the process has become so proficient as to have a self-correcting mechanism. If someone — or something — attempts to interrupt the cycle, there are mechanisms that check the intruder, thus safeguarding the cycle. An example of such a process in two of the families follows.

Some of the self-correcting mechanisms that are present in the case of the six-year-old, mildly retarded boy are these: The mother has declared she has to watch and follow the boy around all the time or he will hurt himself. The suggestion is there. The effect that this statement has is that the boy does hurt himself when alone and this brings mother running, perpetuating the necessity. And since the boy has never been on a picnic

[5]Clinical experiences of the 1971 Workshop come from the clinical data of Eugenia Towner, Dorothy Cravero, Sister Dolores Gencuski, and Marilyn Garin.

without his mother, he is unmanageable by the counselors, thus that myth is perpetuated. But these situations don't have to exist. They have been defined by the system in this manner for a purpose in the system. With the self-correcting mechanism present, it ensures the pattern's survival.

If the uncle doesn't dole out the money in small amounts to the 19-year-old day-care patient the boy will use the large amount to run off and spend all the money. He then is brought back into the system by a collect, long-distance call, and it is necessary again to dole out the money carefully to him, so his future welfare is secure. This is a self-correcting system that reoccurs.

In a system with ingrained, self-defined necessities and self-correcting mechanisms to perpetuate the cycle, there is little chance for change or for growth. On the other hand, signals that people are hurt by these patterns and pathology is growing with the continuing patterns opens the way for therapeutic intervention. The system itself or sometimes a larger system connected with the family might be the referring agent.

In the process of altering necessities, four steps are important to the therapeutic intervention. The first step is to discover the necessity itself, and observe it in process, seeing the pattern in action in order to evaluate what it does for the system.

Second is the challenge to change. People being people are resistant to change, since they are comfortable with the familiar. In pathological situations the resistance is even stronger since the condition has gone beyond comfort to stagnation. Thomas Harris says,

People change because of one of three reasons. First is that they hurt sufficiently. They have beat their heads against the same wall so long that they decide they have had enough. They have invested in the same slot machine so long that they decide they have had enough. Another thing that makes people want to change is a slow type of despair called ennui or boredom. The third thing is the sudden discovery that they can.[6]

And as Wheelis points out, "Usually change — when it occurs at all — follows long and arduous trying."[7] But it can happen. Challenge the necessity with the family. Ask why this has to be. Get their commitment to change this necessity.

Third, once committed to do something about it, have the family explore the other options. Have the family think of the alternatives themselves. Avoid the trap of giving advice or the sewed-up answer. It doesn't work that way. One does not learn to walk by advice from others.

Fourth, after the family members have decided on their new method of action, is putting it into practice and into action. Also use the new

[6]Thomas Harris, MD. *I'm OK — You're OK,* New York, Harper & Row, 1969, Chapter 4, pp. 56.

[7]Allen Wheelis. "Why People Change," *Commentary,* May 1969, pp. 10.

approach until it is refined, and the family is familiar with it. Work out snags in the new method with the family, so they won't slip back into the old necessity pattern.

Of course these four steps are not magic. There is much work and anxiety involved. They do not even work out smoothly all the time. But it is helpful for the therapists to have an outline by which to approach the work.

Necessities can cripple a system can stop growth entirely. In a family, where many people of various ages are living and growing, it is especially important that the family not get steeped in necessity, thus closing the door to growth. The therapist's role is to help show people how to free themselves from their self-defined necessity and put them back on the road toward being in control and being responsible. As Sarte says, "I choose myself not in my being but in my manner of being."[8]

We are our choices.

[8]Jean-Paul Sartre. *The Philosophy of Jean-Paul Sartre,* The Modern Library, New York, Random House, pp. 270, 278.

BIBLIOGRAPHY

Arieti, Silvano. *The Intrapsychic Self,* London, Basic Books, Inc. 1967, pp. 141–143.

Harris, Thomas, MD. *I'm OK — You're OK, New York:* Harper & Row 1969, Chapter 4, pp. 54–64.

Sartre, Jean-Paul. *This Philosophy of Jean-Paul Sartre,* The Modern Library, New York, Random House, pp. 270, 278.

Webster's New International Dictionary, 2nd Edition, G. and C. Meriam Co., Springfield, Mass., 1950, pp. 546–572, 1635, 1636.

Wheelis, Allen. "How People Chance," reprinted from *Commentary,* May, 1969.

Clinical experiences of the 1971 Workshop, from the clinical data of Mrs Eugenia Towner, Dorothy Cravero, Sister Dolores Gencuski, and Marilyn Garin.

6.

One Act Equals One Reaction

Pamela Herriott

"That's the way I've always done it," or "That's the only possible solution" are familiar responses to a family therapist's direction to explore alternatives. Decisions regarding actions in a disturbed family frequently carry the assumption that this is the *one* possible action and all others are unheard of. This selection focuses on the pattern of "one act equals one reaction," explaining how that route becomes set within a family. Suggestions for ways in which the therapist can intervene into that pattern are presented.

From a philosophical point of view, how man gets to be the way he is essentially a question of determinism versus free will. Theories about man fall along the determinism–free will continuum. Rollo May discusses his view.[1]

The danger in the influence of Freudian theory lies in setting up a mechanistic, deterministic view of the personality in the minds of the partially informed public so that people conclude that they are the victims of their instinctual drives and that their only salvation lies in expressing their libido whenever the urge arises.

Frankl notes a similar idea.[2]

Man has been presented as constrained by biological, by psychological, by sociological factors. Inherent human freedom, which obtains in spite of all these constraints, the freedom of the mind in spite of nature, has been overlooked.

May discusses the incongruence of the deterministic view with the goals of therapy, saying that "one of the basic presuppositions in all psychotherapy is that the patient must sooner or later accept responsibility for himself." He also says that "personal determinism, which excuses

[1]Rollo May, *The Art of Counseling*, New York, Abingdon Press, 1967, pp. 48–49.
[2]Viktor Frankl, *The Doctor and the Soul*, New York, Alfred A. Knopf, 1955, p. 23.

him from responsibility, works in the end directly against his regaining mental health."[3]

Existential philosophy does not discredit the influence of heredity and environment on man's development; however, "they" add a third element: decision. They see man as a deciding being — deciding what and who he is. Wheelis in "How People Change" agrees when he says that "we create ourselves."[4]

The particular philosophy a family holds about how man gets to be the way he is has an influence on whether or not they see themselves as being able to have a choice. An example of this is when someone says "it just happened" as contrasted to the statement "I decided" — the former being the deterministic view, and the latter, free will.

Wheelis states that "freedom is the awareness of alternatives and of the ability to choose."[5] In problem solving and decision making there is an obstacle to overcome. A choice or decision is made after the alternative ways for solving the problem are considered. Robert White[6] discusses this in developing his theory of competence. He believes that an individual develops competence in dealing with his environment by exercising his ability to explore and problem solve *on his own*. As he successfully comes to a conclusion, and adds to his repertoire of ways to solve problems, competence is increased. White bases his theory on the idea that problem solving, by itself, is satisfying to the individual.

Rokeach's theory of open and closed mindedness notes that

the basic characteristic that defines the extent to which a person's system is open or closed is the extent to which the individual can receive, evaluate and act on relevant information from the outside on its own intrinsic merits, unencumbered by irrelevant factors in the situation arising from within the person or from the outside.[7]

Looking at the dynamics of closed mindedness, Rokeach notes that a lack of permission to express ambivalent feelings toward the parents leads to anxiety and a narrowing of possibilities for identification with persons outside the family.[8] Wheelis expresses a similar viewpoint when he talks about an unstable identity.[9] A decreased tolerance for conflict increases the need to use "necessity." Necessity is defined as "that range of experience wherein events, course of action, attitudes, decisions are seen as determined by forces outside ourselves which we cannot alter."[10]

[3]Rollo May, op. cit., p. 49.
[4]Allen Wheelis, "How People Change," *Commentary*, May 1969, pp. 9.
[5]Ibid., p. 4.
[6]Robert W. White, "Motivation Reconsidered: The Concept of Competence," *Psychological Review*, 66, 1959, 297–333.
[7]Milton Rokeach, *The Open and Closed Mind*, New York, Basic Books, Inc., 1960, p. 57.
[8]Ibid., pp. 357–365.
[9]Wheelis, op. cit., pp. 3 and 9.
[10]Ibid., p. 10.

Wheelis calls this "psychic housekeeping" — the more issues we have closed, the fewer we have to fret about.[11] An unstable identity has a low tolerance for conflict; therefore, the aim of using "necessity" is to relieve the conflict and also the responsibility for choosing. The risk involved is that the individual is left without resources with which to handle crises. He then reacts within a limited framework, as if he had no choice. It is important to note here that a certain amount of stereotyping or categorizing of responses is necessary. One example, in which immediate categorization is functional, is in an emergency. Otherwise, the much-needed time and energy would be spent in checking out the alternatives and reaching a decision, instead of reacting stereotypically. The other end of the continuum is awareness of all the alternatives. In some cases, awareness of too many alternatives results in an inability to reach a decision. Complete withdrawal or panic might be the outcome. Wheelis notes that adolescence is traditionally the time of greatest freedom.[12] It is also the time of the greatest conflict. One has to just observe an adolescent vehemently espousing an idea at one point, and at another point in a quandary about making a decision because there are just so many choices available.

To clarify the pattern of "one act equals one reaction," it is helpful to define it operationally; that is, to delineate its important aspects in a working definition that can be used to identify this as a pattern. The following definition takes into account the ideas previously mentioned.

1. Determinism as the family philosophy.
2. Decreased self-esteem in individual family members as identified by
   a. Dependence on others to increase self-esteem.
   b. Unstable identity.
   c. Lack of competence in problem-solving.
3. Decreased tolerance for conflict.
4. Obstacle or problem (stimulus).
5. Increase in tension — conflict.
6. Lack of awareness of alternatives producing a feeling of "no choice" — "necessity."
7. One fixed response for that stimulus.
8. Action in a fixed way.
9. Decrease in tension — conflict.

The important concepts in this definition are (1) the dependence on others for self-esteem and identity and (2) the decreased tolerance for conflict. These "lock" the family members into a set pattern of behaving and

[11]Wheelis, op. cit., p. 9.
[12]Ibid., p. 9.

present exploration of alternatives. An example of this is taken from an interview with a marital dyad. At this point in the interview they were discussing their decision to get married.

Husband: The only trouble was that she was Catholic and I was Protestant.

Therapist: How did you solve that problem?

H: Well she said she wouldn't marry me because I was Protestant. I said I guess I can fix that so the next Tuesday I went to see the priest. I didn't let her know.

T: So you decided this yourself. How did you make that decision?

H: It wasn't very hard.

Wife: This girl always has to know why we do things.

H: It wasn't very hard.

W: Why to everything (overlapping H's comments).

H: . . . if you love somebody enough — nothing's in your way. I felt it was worthwhile.

W: Well his folks were Baptist, but he didn't really believe in it.

H: I was never baptised in any church at the time so it wasn't hard for me to change to Catholic.

T: I'm wondering what alternatives you saw at that point.

H: None.

T: So you saw becoming a Catholic as the only alternative.

H: Yes.

W: It wasn't the only thing you could have done.

H: I didn't want to lose her and I thought this was the only way that she and I could ever get together — get along, and I wasn't going to spoil her religion. I know I didn't have any.

T: So you thought that you would have to change to marry her.

H: Yes.

T: (to W) You mentioned that there were other alternatives.

W: It wasn't strictly required. A Protestant and a Catholic can get married — if we wanted to.

H: Yeah but that was my idea myself.

T: What did you think about it when he told you?

W: I was glad it was this way, then the children don't have any conflict.

H: Most of my friends were Catholic — French.

T: I was wondering — when you said it wouldn't have been necessary for him to change to marry you. He had a different idea about that — he thought that the only way he could marry you was to become a Catholic.

W: No I don't mean — I mean really I didn't feel as if I wanted to marry him — anybody different from me. There's a conflict if you're not the same.

This example meets the criteria for the pattern "one act equals one reaction." The decreased tolerance for conflict was explicitly stated by the wife, and the husband illustrated well the "feeling of no choice" when he stated that it was the only way they could get along.

How therapeutic intervention into this pattern might be managed is suggested by Wheelis.[13]

Since freedom depends upon awareness, psychotherapy may, by extending awareness, create freedom. When in therapy a life story of drift and constraint is reworked to expose alternatives for crucial courses of action, asking always "Why did you do that?," attaching doubt to every explanation which is cast in the form of necessary reaction to antecedent cause, always reminding the patient that "Even so . . . it was possible to have acted otherwise" — in all this one is rewriting the past, is taking the story of a life which was experienced as shaped by circumstances and which was recounted as such, and retelling it in terms of choice and responsibility. And insofar as it may come to seem credible to rewrite one's life in terms of ignored choice, to assume responsibility retrospectively for what one has done and so has become, it will be possible likewise to see alternatives in the present. . . .

By his exploration into the alternatives, the therapist teaches the individual family members that they do have a choice. The therapist also in his exploration goes through the problem-solving steps with the family. In this way, by his modeling behavior, the individual members are able to increase their competence in solving problems.

Haley discusses the strategy of the therapeutic paradoxical injunction as an effective means to initiate change.[14] Operationally defined, it is:

1. An intense relationship (psychotherapeutic situation).
   a. High degree of survival value.
   b. Defined as one where change is to take place.
2. An injunction (order) is given by the therapist.
   a. Encouraging-reinforcing the behavior that is expected to change.

[13]Wheelis, op. cit., p. 14.
[14]Jay Haley, *Strategies of Psychotherapy*, New York, Grune and Stratton, Inc., 1963, pp. 179–191.

3. There follows an "illustion of choice."
   a. to obey the injunction — voluntary control of the behavior.
   b. To disobey the injunction — undesirable behavior ceases.
4. There is blockage of escape from the therapeutic situation by
   a. Withdrawal or
   b. Commenting on the "illusion of choice."
5. This forces the individuals to step outside their usual frame of behaving; that is, changed if he does and changed if he does not.

Wheelis notes that "we are what we do"[15]; therefore, in order to change what we are we have to change what we do. This view is congruent with the therapeutic-paradoxical injunction, since it is behavior that is the focus.

Intervention must begin almost immediately, because frequently families are seen on a short-term basis, and it is necessary to introduce a new way of looking at things quickly. When the therapist hears a pattern of fixed response, work can begin at that moment, focusing on examination of alternatives.

[15]Wheelis, op. cit., p. 3.

BIBLIOGRAPHY

Frankl, Viktor. *The Doctor and the Soul,* New York, Alfred A. Knopf, 1955, pp. 1–26.

Haley, Jay. *Strategies of Psychotherapy,* New York, Grune and Stratton, Inc., 1963, pp. 179–191.

May, Rollo. *The Art of Counseling,* New York, Abingdon Press, 1967, pp. 44–97.

Rokeach, Milton. *The Open and Closed Mind,* New York, Basic Books, Inc., 1960.

Rokeach, Milton. *Beliefs, Attitudes and Values: A Theory of Organization and Change,* San Francisco: Jossey-Bass, Inc., Publishers, 1968. (Background information only.)

Wheelis, Allen. "How People Change," *Commentary,* May 1969, pp. 1–19.

White, Robert W. "Motivation Reconsidered: The Concept of Competence," *Psychological Review, 66,* 1959, 297–333.

7.

Decision-Making Process in a Marital Dyad

Sharon Pecha

The process of decision making within a family system is vitally important to the adequate functioning of the system. This selection explores some of the ways that decisions are often made within families and focuses on a rational type of decision making. A clinical example of a marital dyad is presented. This couple's lack of ability to make decisions adequately within their family system has resulted in the need for therapeutic intervention. Some therapeutic approaches have been made with the couple and are discussed here.

Decision making is a dynamic process involving conflict and harmonization. Family members are faced with the necessity or desire to choose between two or more alternatives of varied nature in various situations and in some way they make a choice of one alternative. Webster defines decision as "an act or process of arriving at a solution that ends uncertainty or dispute about."[1]

The family is a social system made up of family member subsystems and itself functioning as a subsystem within the larger systems of society.

For human social systems, Bredemeier says there are three critical processes for system survival. The system must: (1) adapt to its environments; (2) integrate its parts (roles and collectivities composed of roles); and (3) decide on the modes of carrying out and the resources to be allocated to the first two processes.[2]

There are four basic things that must be done by a social system in order to adapt to its environment. These four things are: "obtain matter;

---

[1]*Webster's Seventh New Collegiate Dictionary,* Springfield, Mass., G. & C. Merriam Co., 1963, p. 214.

[2]Shirley A. Smoyak, "Toward Understanding Nursing Situations: A Transaction Paradigm," *Nursing Research,* **18**:5, September-October 1969, 407. (Smoyak quoting Bredemeier, unpublished manuscript.)

nonhuman energy, information and human energy (or services) from the environment; dispose of some of them to the environment; contain some of them in the environment (i.e., prevent them from entering the system); and retain some of them in itself (i.e., prevent their moving from the system to the environment."[3] The process of decision making within the family is, therefore, vitally important to the ability of the family to continue functioning as an integral system. It determines *how* adaptation will be managed.

More specifically in terms of a group such as the family, Turner says, "By group decision making we mean a process directed toward unambivalent group assent and commitment to a course of action or inaction. The ideas of assent and commitment serve to distinguish group decision from the decision and action of an individual member."[4]

There are several ways of making decisions within the family group, and these differ in the kind and amount of assent or commitment from the individuals involved. A reasonable process of making decisions allows the exploration of available alternatives by individual members within the group. After members feel they have an understanding of the alternatives, they can negotiate among themselves about the choice they will make. Age and power differences determine the likelihood that democracy will or will not be allowed as a mode.

The ideal image of decision making is one in which the initial differences of viewpoint are eliminated through discussion until there is eventual agreement. The result is a decision to which all give equal assent and all feel equally committed without private reservation or personal resentment. A decision of this kind is known as consensus. It is not so frequent in the family as romance would have it.[5]

The more common kind of decision process in which the decision is made without assent from all family members is termed by Turner as

accommodation; agreement is achieved by the adjustment of some or all of the members to the irreconcilability of their views. The accommodation may be achieved amiably or with bitterness. An accommodation is always an agreement to disagree, to adopt a common decision in the face of recognized and unreconciled private desires.[6]

This kind of decision making often involves bargaining among all family members, or as we shall consider later, between the marital dyad. Lederer and Jackson discuss the largely unconscious bargaining that occurs regularly in marriage and they call this system of behavioral responses the *quid pro quo*.

[3]Ibid., p. 407 (Smoyak quoting Bredemeier, unpublished manuscript).
[4]Ralph H. Turner, *Family Interaction,* New York, Wiley, 1970, p. 97.
[5]Ibid., p. 98.
[6]Ibid.

Quid pro quo *literally means "something for something." In the mar-riage process, it means that if you do so-and-so, then I automatically will respond with such-and-such. The* quid pro quo *is largely unconscious. Marital rules and interactions often exist in an evenly working fashion without either spouse's being aware of their presence.*[7]

These rules of *quid pro quo* may come into conscious awareness at the time of a family decision. For instance, family members may consciously decide to agree on a certain matter even though one or more of them may disagree with the choice that is made. The full agreement does not only include the choice made, but also an arrangement for one or some of the members to receive something in exchange for the concession they have made to the others.

A further look at decisions that are reached by consensus or accommo-dation leads to a consideration of the values involved in the process. Turner describes three ways in which an individual's values can undergo change so that conclusions can be reached by the group. First, involves the introduction of a new proposal that influences the disparity and is in agreement to the member's values. Second, a different value that is in agreement with the dissenting members' values may be applied to the disagreement so that it is then seen in a new light. Third, some members may change their image of the decision and its effects perhaps through increased understanding of the effects. Therefore, values are closely involved with the decision process, and the greater the agreement among individuals about values the greater the chance for consensual agreements.[8]

The more extensive the common values of family members, the less likelihood there is for disagreement and for resulting dominance by one or several family members who are continually identified with the decisions that are made. This likelihood also is lessened when family members have a clear understanding of each other's values.

Through consensus or accommodation the family makes a choice of one of the available alternatives and completes a rational decision making process. Assent and commitment are elements that distinguish a group decision from an individual decision. The family members may actively agree to the irrevocability of assent."[9] In the group some members may view the decision as that of some other members and, therefore, will not feel commitment to the decision. The more consent of agreement that is felt by family members the more commitment each one feels to the decision.

[7]William J. Lederer and Don J. Jackson, *The Mirages of Marriage,* New York, W. W. Norton & Company, 1968, pp. 178, 184.
[8]Turner, pp. 99-100.
[9]Ibid., p. 98.

The transactions between family members that occur during the process of decision making can be described in terms of various modes. "Transactions between systems consist of efforts of one to induce compliance while the other resists or does not resist the effort in varying degrees."[10] The tactics employed in these transactions have been classified by Bredemeier into five major types: coercion or force, bargaining or marketing, legal-bureaucratic, team-cooperative, and gemeinschaft. These five modes can be described by the answer each type gives to the ever-present question, "Why should I?" asked by the one expected to conform to the demand.[11] In decision making the specific question is, "Why should I agree to the particular decision?" Other questions besides "Why?" include "*How* shall the decision be made?" and "*What* shall be decided?" These mode types are helpful in understanding the family interactions in the decision making process.

The answers of each type to "Why should I?" are the following. In the bargaining mode the answer is, "Because doing so will bring a more valued *quid pro quo* than not doing so."[12] The objective is to maximize profit and minimize costs. The legal-bureaucratic mode answers, "Because it is your duty.[13] This mode is most often effective when the participants are both part of a larger system of rules and enforcements. Team-cooperative gives, as the reason, "Because doing so will facilitate the requesting system's contribution to a collective goal.[14] The gemeinschaft mode is based on the adapting system seeing itself as particularly significant to the other for reasons of some status quality such as a friend or spouse and answers, "Why should I?" with, "Because it will make the other better off."[15] The coercive mode uses such tactics as force, fraud, or deception.[16]

Each family member involved in the decision making process has an expectation of the type of mode that should be employed in making the decision. If each participant expects the same mode, conformity is achieved, and they will proceed in the same mode to make the required decision. If they are not in agreement, one will perceive the other with various kinds of dissatisfaction depending on the modes expected by each person. For instance, if the husband expects his wife to agree with him out of love and care for him (gemeinschaft mode), he will be disappointed and feel she is cold and uncaring if she agrees with him because she feels it is her duty to do so (legal-bureaucratic mode). These modes will be illustrated further in the particular family that will be discussed later.

---

[10]Smoyak, p. 408.
[11]Ibid., p. 408 (Smoyak quoting Bredemeier, unpublished manuscript).
[12]Ibid., p. 408 (Smoyak quoting Bredemeier, unpublished manuscript).
[13]Ibid.
[14]Ibid., p. 409.
[15]Ibid.
[16]Ibid.

After the family has made a choice, they are likely to experience a phase of regret about the decision. Studies have been carried out by Festinger and Walster to the "conclusion that at least under some conditions there is a measurable period of post-decision regret. Indirect evidence of this, in the form of post-decision reversal of choice, was obtained in the Festinger and Walster experiment, and very direct evidence was obtained in the Walster experiment."[17] In the regret phase after a decision is made, the individual

is struck by the fact that by choosing one alternative, he has lost all the good qualities of the other. He begins to doubt whether he made the right decision, and he sometimes regrets that he made the one he did. This usually lasts for only a brief time, but during this period, he actually has a tendency to decrease his evaluation of the alternative he chose and to increase the other one. However, the regret phase soon passes, dissonance reduction occurs, and the chosen alternative ends up valued higher than it was before and the unchosen one ends up valued lower.[18]

These phases of post-decision regret and then dissonance reduction, as have been studied in individual decision making, are also present in individuals when family decisions have been made because they must go along with the decision that is made and must give up whatever qualities they see as part of the choice not taken. Regret is likely to be greater when some members do not agree with the final group decision.

Knowledge that one or some alternatives must be decided against may well be a retarding factor in an individual's or family's willingness to actively make decisions. "Decisions are dependent upon a person's ability to confine himself to the choice made and to renounce the possibilities which are inherent in the other alternatives. The ability to commit oneself is based on the mobilization of all resources for a given task."[19] The family members may be unable to mobilize their forces in one choice and in doing so refuse to make a decision.

Many situations occur within families in which no conclusion is reached by the family group. The outcome of these situations are then decided by external events. For instance, the members may not be able to decide between several kinds of entertainment until it is too late to attend any. *What all such events have in common is that agreement is by the absence of dissent rather than by active assent, and, more important, commitment is by the course of events rather than by acceptance. Such decisions are made in fact rather than in words but in a context of events*

[17]Leon Festinger, *Conflict, Decision, and Dissonance*, Stanford, California, Stanford University Press, 1964, p. 127.
[18]Jonathan L. Freedman, J. Merrill Carlsmith, and David O. Sears, *Social Psychology*, Englewood Cliffs, New Jersey, Prentice-Hall, Inc., 1970, pp. 358-359.
[19]Jurgen Ruesch, *Therapeutic Communication*, New York, W. W. Norton & Company, 1961, p. 329.

such that members of the group find themselves committed. Consequently we borrow a term from law to designate these as de facto decisions.[20]

In addition to the above possibilities in decision making a family may choose a person outside the family for consultation about family decisions. In doing so they may avoid making their own decisions but, frequently, are unhappy with the advice they receive and focus on their disagreement with the outside party.

When the family system becomes unable to adequately make decisions stress is felt throughout the system. As Smoyak points out,

systems cannot operate without a decision making part functioning so as to insure that rules will be followed. With no centralized decision maker operating, it is highly unlikely that human social systems will function in concert.[21]

Mr. and Mrs. D. are an example of a family who are experiencing stress within their marital system resulting from inability to successfully decide who will make which decisions. Mr. D., age 61, has a bachelor's degree in economics, was in the army for 9 years, and has been retired with civil service and veteran's pensions for the past 10 years. From the age of 24 he has experienced intermittent episodes of "mental illness" that seem to have been characterized by what he calls a voice impediment (speaking in a broken voice), nervousness, and depression. These epidsodes were accompanied by admissions to mental hospitals.

At age 52, he married Mrs. D. who was then 49. She had been working as a civil service bookkeeper for 15 years. During 11 years of that period she had one serious boyfriend whom she reportedly wanted to marry but did not because she had learned he was already married. This boyfriend introduced her to Mr. D. whom she married after a courtship of one-and-a-half years. Mrs. D. knew her husband's history of mental illness, but says she never considered him to be sick. She felt he needed security and love and that he seemed to be calmer when he was around her.

Before the marriage the couple agreed on a Dutch treat arrangement that they describe in the following manner: Mrs. D. would continue to work and bring in her income while Mr. D. would contribute his pension and would do all of the housework that would be worth a certain amount of money. It was agreed that this arrangement would result in equal mometary input by each. This arrangement was satisfactory not only from the financial aspect but also in respect to adequately filling time with activity and reportedly worked well until three years ago when Mrs. D. retired, and the couple moved 1500 miles from their home. Since that time there have been frequent, minor difficulties mostly around decisions about spending money and time. The crisis that brought Mr. D. to the

[20]Turner, pp. 99-100.
[21]Smoyak, p. 410.

Veterans Hospital, Psychiatric Unit was the purchasing of a sidewalk and a pursuant argument with Mrs. D. about the decision to buy the sidewalk.

A continuing problem for Mr. and Mrs. D. has centered around the spending of money. The following dialogue explains part of the trouble.

Mrs. D.: I think spending of money should be mutual regardless of what source, but the basic difference here is that I am very conservative and I will do without things even if there is money in the bank.

Mr. D.: What do you do without?

Mrs. D.: Clothing — I could use more clothes, more shoes.

Mr. D.: Have I ever vetoed any purchase you've ever made?

Mrs. D.: Oh no! This is the difference. Now I will be conservative and not buy and he'll say "buy two" regardless of where the money comes from.

Mr. D.: I'm spending well within my income — under my income.

Mr. and Mrs. D. are expressing different values that influence the way money is spent. Although they would like to confer and agree on expenditures, they cannot because they differ in the basic value each places on spending and saving money. The resulting commitment they will have to a decision will be conditional because of their value differences.

Another problem lies in the area of who does the decision making in which areas of spending. Mr. D. would like to consult his wife about purchases but would like to have the final word about certain things, particularly his clothing. The following is an example.

Mr. D.: I would like to tell her I need a shirt and she should just accept that because I know more about my clothing than she does — these are personal items of mine.

Mrs. D.: Well, I would like to be able to agree that he did need it.

Mr. D.:   Well, why don't you?

Therapist: So you, Mrs. D., want a voice in the purchase?

Mrs. D.: Yea.

Mr. D.: Oh, yes — she should have a voice in it! But since the amount involved is so small, I don't think I should give up my right to buy a shirt. I think I should be able to override her veto. And, if she wants to buy something she should be able to override my veto which she wouldn't get anyway. I don't veto anything she wants. One person has to have the right to make the final decision. If it is her clothing I should only have the right to suggest to her. I think the same should apply to me where small amounts of money are involved, especially clothing. However, if larger amounts of money are involved, we should talk about it and decide, like furniture. Anything over $5 or $10.

Therapist: How do you feel about this, Mrs. D.?

Mrs. D.: He doesn't have to stop me from buying something because he knows in advance I don't buy something unless it's something I absolutely need. I think almost everything should be decided by both people.

Mr. D.: No, see we disagree.

The problematic decision, and one that Mr. and Mrs. D. refuse to make, is who should make which decisions about which purchases. The result is that events that usually occur in a store are frequently the deciding factor and leave both persons feeling they have been taken advantage of.

Further difficulty lies in the modes of transaction each of the partners feels should be used in making decisions. Recently the couple decided to go for a short ride. Mr. D. invited his wife because he thought it would be a pleasant experience. Mrs. D. agreed, feeling that she should take the time and go with her husband. When Mr. D. learned about his wife's motivation, he became irritated and said there had been no use going if she didn't want to. He told her that he would rather not have her go with him if she felt she had to do it. He expected a gemeinschaft mode of transaction when she was interacting in a legal-bureaucratic mode.

An understanding of each person's expectations for the mode of transaction to be used in helpful in making a therapeutic intervention. In another decision about the structuring of time Mr. and Mrs. D. were able to come to an agreement that was suggested by the therapist where in a legal-bureaucratic mode Mr. D. took it as his duty to allow Mrs. D. a certain amount of time for individual activities. Mrs. D. then responded in the gemeinschaft mode to him by spending time with him out of gratitude for her individual time. Each received what he desired in a manner that each desired.

The primary therapeutic intervention was directed toward exploration with Mr. and Mrs. D. of the decisions they make and the decision making process they use. They were able to give many reasons about why they should make various decisions but had considerable difficulty focusing on the manner in which they did the deciding. They were set in their patterns of trying to convince each other of their own ideas to the point that they could not see how they were going about making decisions. Lederer and Jackson compare some marital couples to a computer that has been incorrectly programmed and can be corrected only by a human being changing the program. "The computer itself does not observe its own mistakes; neither do most married couples see their own pattern; they are caught up within the system and are not able to look at themselves from a vantage point outside."[22]

[22]Lederer and Jackson, p. 186.

By taking a new look at their system processes with the therapist's direction, Mr. and Mrs. D. were able to begin considering how they actually go about making decisions. When the different kinds of decision making processes were pointed out by the therapist, Mrs. D. responded by saying, "Yes, that is the way it happens," and agreed that coming to some definite agreement was more desirable then allowing de facto decisions to be made.

Alternate modes of transaction were suggested as possibilities that Mr. and Mrs. D. might want to consider and use in making decisions. The possibility of making bargains about the activities that they want to share and others that they prefer to do alone was explored. Additional consideration of who should be in charge of what areas was also explored along with the ways they can decide about which of them has what power in which areas of family decisions.

This selection described a rational decision making process that can be used by a family in order to function as an integral system. Factors that influence the process were discussed. The difficulties in making decisions in a marital dyad were explored, and techniques of therapeutic intervention with this couple were suggested.

BIBLIOGRAPHY

Festinger, Leon. *Conflict, Decision, and Dissonance,* Stanford, California, Stanford University Press, 1964.

Freedman, Jonathan L., J. Merrill Carlsmith, and David O. Sears. *Social Psychology,* Englewood Cliffs, New Jersey, Prentice-Hall, Inc., 1970.

Lederer, William J. and Don D. Jackson. *The Mirages of Marriage,* New York, W. W. Norton & Company, 1968.

Ruesch, Jurgen. *Therapeutic Communication,* New York, W. W. Norton & Company, 1961.

Smoyak, Shirley A. "Toward Understanding Nursing Situations: A Transaction Paradigm," *Nursing Research,* **18:** 5, September-October, 1969, 405-411.

Turner, Ralph H. *Family Interaction,* New York, 1970.

Websters's Seventh New Collegiate Dictionary, Springfield, Massachusetts, G. & C. Merriam Company, 1963.

8.

New Families, New Marriages

Gwen Gorman

This selection reviews some of the differences and similarities of marital dyads as they are presented in new families and new marriages. Areas included are reasons for marriage, cultural considerations, decision-making schemes, communication patterns, establishment of rules, resolution of disagreements, role expectations, system values, and standards of socialization. Particular emphasis has been placed on the nursing intervention in the areas concerned with the infringement of a subsystem into an established system.

REVIEW OF LITERATURE FOR SOCIOLOGICAL
ASPECTS OF MARITAL ADJUSTMENT

Approximately 400,000 people are divorced annually[1] in the United States. The subsequent remarriage of parents results in many adjustments for the parents and children. Family therapists may find many of the situations in the new family slightly different from problems in "old" families.

New families consist of the marital dyad, newly married, with one or both spouses having at least one unmarried offspring from a previous marriage. The term "newly married" as used in relation to families will include the last seven years. A new marriage refers to a marital dyad having entered into marriage without children.

The newly formed families included in this clinical study were new in the sense that the children had been added to the marital dyad in the last four months. They will be referred to throughout the paper as quasiadults. They varied in age from 18 to 27 years.

[1]William J. Lederer and Don D. Jackson, *The Mirages of Marriage*, New York, W. W. Norton & Company, Inc., 1968, p. 15.

REASONS FOR MARRIAGE

Many people in the Unived States may assume that "love" is the basis for marriage; however, Lederer and Jackson list this idea as "false assumption" number one,

People marry because they love each other. They like to think of themselves as being in love; however, by and large the emotion they interpret as love is in reality some other emotion — often a strong sex drive, fear, or a hunger for approval.

They also list the following reasons for marriage.

"Because society expects it of them."

"Pressures and the maneuverings' of parents often push their children into premature and careless marriage."

"Loneliness often drives people into marriage."

"Many people are fearful concerning their economic future."

"Individuals marry because of an unconscious desire to improve themselves."

"Many marriages are motivated by neuroses."

"Some people miss their father or mother and cannot live without a parental symbol."[2]

Horney adds that "some quality in the partner . . . corresponds to some . . . expectation"[3] that the individual had of the marital partner prior to marriage.

It is generally accepted in society that ethnic background and religion may have some influence on a marital partner. The manner in mate selection is generally believed to be consistent for first and second marriages. The felt necessity for finding an appropriate parent for an offspring may influence the selection process.

CULTURAL CONSIDERATION

Each culture carries with it a set of symbols and may place different interpretations on these symbols. This may lead to misunderstandings for the new relationships if they have crossed cultures.

Bredemeier and Stephenson describe the "differences in cultures are those that tell people what to perceive and those that tell them how to respond to what they perceive." They also mention that what may be morally required in one culture may be morally prohibited in another. In

[2]Ibid., pp. 42–45.
[3]Karen Horney, *Feminine Psychology,* New York, W. W. Norton & Co., Inc., 1967, p. 122.

addition they mention that "some analysis of culture and personality have suggested the basic personality traits themselves influence the nature of culture and set the limits within which change or alterations of the cultural pattern takes place."[4]

On the basis of the above it is easily seen that marriages across cultures will require a great deal of compromise and adjustment for each of the marital partners. This adjustment would be necessary for any couple; however, with the additional family members involved with new families, the number of adjustments may be in proportion to the number of people involved.

DECISION-MAKING SCHEMES

Individuals differ in their methods of making decisions. Some individuals will use the legal-bureaucratic method, which calls on an individual's duty to respond to a request. Some may use bargaining as a means of decision making. The gemeinschaft method is still another that calls on the individual to respond as a matter of family system obligation. A final method is the team-cooperative approach whereby those involved work for the good of all involved.[5]

Some of the decision-making schemes are more in harmony than other combinations. The greatest cohesiveness would naturally be assumed with those marital couples who used the same method of decision making.

While similarities may exist with marital couples of both categories (new marriages and new families), the conflict increases in direct proportion to the differences in the number of people involved and to their previous orientation to decision-making schemes. The previous orientation to decision making would be a major consideration for quasiadults coming into the family.

One example of this type of disharmony is cited in a clinical session:[6]

Mother: I like to be told what you are thinking, I cannot second guess. Tell me in a straightforward way so I can understand.

Son: I am an emotional person. I am more of an emotional person than a thinker.

In this case the mother was a legal-bureaucratic decision maker, and the son used the gemeinschaft method of decision making. A great deal of

[4]Harry C. Bredemeier and Richard Stephenson, *The Analysis of Social Systems,* New York, Holt, Rinehart and Winston, Inc., 1965, pp. 2, 11, 84.
[5]Shirley Smoyak, "Toward Understanding Nursing Situations: A Transaction Paradigm," *Nursing Research,* **18:**5, September-October 1969
[6]Appreciation and credit is given to Nellie Rodgers and Edith McRae, who participated in and supplied data to the Advanced Workshop in Psychiatric Nursing Skills.

compromise is necessary to produce harmony in interacting when the new family members have used opposing styles in their past families.

COMMUNICATION PATTERNS

A primary objective of communication is for both sender and receiver to share mutual meaning in the same message. According to Satir the word "communication" can mean "interaction" or "transaction." "Communication" also includes all those symbols and clues used by persons in giving and receiving meaning.[7] Vital information is received in two basic ways:

We ask for verbal responses.

We also observe nonverbal behavior.[8]

Some of the difficulties posed by simple verbal communication are:

1. The same word can have different meanings, different denotations.

2. The same word can have different connotations.

3. Words themselves are often unclear.[9]

The therapist will often use tone, tension, and voice frequency for additional input to interpret and understand what the client is saying. People familiar with one another will frequently know by mannerisms, eye movement, grimacing, quickness of movements or their absence and the opinions, feelings, inferences, or moods of one another.

Unfamiliarity between people means a person must seek verbal clarification or confirmation to many words or phrases that are unclear. Frequently, marital pairs will reveal during therapy that the meaning of words exchanged at some time previously has suddenly become clear. An example of one such situation was:

Wife: I asked him (husband) in an angry tone of voice if he were giving away all that merchandise to that man.

Husband: Yes, and that was something we had previously agreed upon, so I couldn't understand why you were so mad.

The husband subsequently decided that if his wife was always changing her mind about what they had decided on and she became angry about it — it must be impossible to please her. He would just quit the business and give up. It was revealed in counseling sessions that the true meaning of

[7]Virginia Satir, *Conjoint Family Therapy,* Palo Alto, California, Science and Behavior Books Inc., 1967, p. 63.

[8]*Ibid.,* p. 64.

[9]*Ibid.,* pp. 64–65.

the sentence had referred to the man and a personal dislike for him and had nothing to do with the decision to give the merchandise away. Such clarifications are frequently corrected in therapy sessions.

Misinterpretations of what was said or not said can be especially troublesome to newlyweds of both categories. In this way they are similar. The difference exists with the addition of each person to the system. The greater the number of interpersonal communications between more people the greater the number of difficulties in decoding the messages.

Patterns that have been previously established between a part of the family, that is, parent and offspring must be redirected into new patterns of communication. The new system must establish its own patterns. This may present itself with some difficulty to the "newcomer," that is, the new spouse.

ESTABLISHING RULES

Haley notes that

each situation that a newly married couple meets must be dealt with by establishing explicit or implicit rules to follow . . . Marital conflict centers in (a) disagreements about the rules for living together, (b) disagreements about who is to set those rules, and (c) attempts to enforce rules which are incompatible with each other. A further area of conflict for a couple occurs if there is an incompatibility between (a) the metarules they establish for resolving disagreements about rules, and (b) the rules themselves. It is important to note that the couple cannot avoid establishing these rules: whenever they complete a transaction, a rule is being established.[10]

Such rules usually worked out between the spouses. These rules are then established for the children and enforced by the parents.

The difficulty in new families comes about when quasiadults enter the family and rules must be defined for them that are consistent with their age and stage of development. Such confusion over the rules is reflected in the statement of one father who stated during a session:

They have been out in the armed services and it's different when they come back.

Another parent stated.

They have their own lives to live, they have to break away from the apron strings and live their own lives more or less.

Such statements reflect uncertainty on the part of the parents as to what rules they can expect the quasiadult to follow. What rules are reasonable for their system?

[10]Jay Haley, *Strategies of Psychotherapy*, New York, Grune and Stratton, 1963, pp. 123, 125, 128.

Since some system rules are implicit expectations, these rules sometimes become the most troublesome. An example of such a rule can be noted in the following interview:

Therapist: How could this misunderstanding have been prevented?

Father: Well, T., could change and be more like us.

At this point the therapist must assist the system in identifying what the expectations are within the system.

All marital dyads must establish rules between themselves, but it is only with new families that extensions of the rules must be considered to encompass subsystems. New families must determine the amount of authority, responsibility, and freedom it will allow each family member. These determinations must be made in a relatively short span of time instead of with the aging and developmental process.

RESOLUTIONS OF DISAGREEMENTS

Disagreements and arguments are sometimes helpful to a marriage, and at other times they may hurt the marital dyad if they are unresolved. Lederer and Jackson state, "vigorously and uneqivocally that bargaining is an essential part of the workable marriage."[11] Promoting bargaining on an open basis is frequently a transaction encouraged by the family therapist. The establishment of the first bargain may quite likely take an entire session. After the system has caught on to the operation of open bargaining it can become a helpful means of compromise. Consider the third session of bargaining in the following therapy session:

Wife: I am unhappy because you ask for catsup on your steak. It is an insult to my cooking.

Husband: It shouldn't be, I just happen to like the taste of catsup on steak.

Wife: If you want catsup, why didn't you get up and get it and not ask me for it.

Husband: Why do you have to answer me as if I ask for something terrible?

Therapist: How about some bargaining?

Wife: Okay, I'll not say anything if he gets up and gets his own catsup.

Bargaining is best done on an action-for-action basis, usually between the marital dyad. Generally, it is not appropriate for the children. Bargaining

[11]Lederer and Jackson, p. 272.

may be considered for problematic areas between quasiadults and the marital dyad, as in the following situation:

Mother: I dislike T. spending all day in his room watching television. I wish he would get out and do something.

T.: I wouldn't mind going out bowling once in awhile if she wouldn't expect me to play bridge with her club.

A bargain then ensued whereby T. would go bowling instead of being expected to play bridge.

ROLES AND EXPECTATIONS

The role of wife/husband does not contain the dimensions that wife-mother/husband-father does. Bredemeier and Stephenson define roles in terms of

any given status in a particular systems involves the person in interaction with a number of persons in other statuses. The actual acting out of a status in interaction with another status-occupant we call a role.[12]

While culture dictates some of the role involvements of husband-wife and mother-father, it is the individuals who must accept the role and its obligations. It is also important to note that a role requires two persons to play a role. A woman cannot be a mother without a child. She cannot be a wife without a husband.

For the new marriage, each partner anticipates immediately assuming their ideal roles and having the opportunity to become adjusted to the husband/wife role before adding the roles of father/mother. In new families the combination of roles leads to greater and quicker change if successful adjustment takes place in a minimum of time. Change usually produces anxiety; therefore, new families can usually expect more unrest and noise in the adjustment period. Since the quasiadults have been exposed to one set of expectations from a former parent, the adjustment of new family expectations between child and stepparent can result in more change. Some change can be positive. Consider the statements made by a stepson:

Stepson: I can talk to my step Mother where I couldn't my real Mother. I've moved up from the gutter to the sidewalk.

Other problems concern how parents, unfamiliar with the growth and development processes of their stepchildren, react and cope with unfamiliar problems.

[12]Bredemeier and Stephenson, The *Analysis of Social Systems,* New York, Holt, Rinehart and Winston, Inc., 1965, p. 38.

ESTABLISHMENT OF SYSTEM OF VALUES

Each person enters a system with a set of values. If the values are similar in the marital dyad very little readjustment will be needed. If spouse comes with a diversity of values a new system will need to be devised. This may be done through a scheme of priority and classification of values.

New marriages have only the marital dyad to cope with in establishing a new standard of values.

New families may be different in that at least part of the value system will have been established in a prior home or community environment. The number of changes will increase in proportion to the number of siblings added to the family. New family systems may establish their values through decision making schemes or through establishment of rules and regulations.

ACCEPTED STANDARDS OF SOCIALIZATION

The one area of immediate attention peculiar to the new family is the establishment of accepted standards of socialization for offspring. McCandless describes
socialization as both process and product. One dimension listed is the generally accepted ways of behaving within the effective culture; and limits beyond which behavior is not permitted.[13]
Many of the new marital dyad values and cultural standards will effect the socialization process of the children. The basic socialization processes are frequently established by the time adolescence is complete. Since socialization is established by "an approving sort of general acceptance — the broadest kind of noncontingent reinforcement seems to be essential for positive self-esteem to develop,"[14] it is conceivable that development of socialization may have been retarded in a troubled family. If the basic socialization patterns have been established before the new family was established and the past socialization patterns emerge as unacceptable to the new parent, a noise can be expected within the new system.

Such statements as the following can be heard in therapy sessions.

Mother: You can teach a child the difference in right and wrong and other things, for them to be helpful when they are out on their own, but what can I teach them now?

[13]Ibid., pp. 352–354.
[14]Ibid. p. 354.

Mother: Why doesn't he get out and meet somebody. I wish he would get married and have some grandchildren for me.

These statements reflect the uncertainty of parents in the new families on what to do with their quasiadult children.

NURSING INTERVENTION FOR NEW FAMILIES

Infringement of subsystems on established systems is a frequent reason for beginning family therapy.

Coalitions in families are most healthy when they are within the appropriate power levels. Children in healthy families grow up with the concept that parents are going to stick together. When one parent, through divorce or death of a spouse, assumes the sole responsibility for the family, frequently the oldest child will assume some of the burden of the missing parent. A coalition will frequently be seen between the parent and the oldest child. This type of coalition can then become troublesome to displaced offspring when new families are formed. When the marriage occurs there is a tendency for the jealousy or hostility to occur toward the new parent who is taking the quasiadult or offsprings' place beside the natural parent. The change and restructuring of coalitions can be painful and noisy. The coalitions may be very difficult to break if the natural parent has been child oriented throughout the life of the offspring. The therapist should encourage and support any threads of coalitions within the power levels. Friedman, Boszormenyi-Nagy, and Jungreis also mention that "the emergence of any single event (e.g., a heated discussion) can significantly change (a) an individual member's habitual behavior, (b) the nature of the dyadic or subgroup interactional patterns (coalition, etc.) and, (c) the overall style of the entire family."[15]

The coalition may exist because the natural parent feels a great burden for the currently unacceptable behavior of the offspring by a previous marriage. The offspring or quasiadult may need help from the dyad in the form of emotional support, assistance with the finishing of the socialization processes never completed during adolescence or he may need some honest feedback to the unacceptable behavior he is exhibiting. If the burden on the natural parent becomes too great it results in anxiety and a dysfunctional relationship between the quasiadults and the parent.

The therapist may be of assistance in reinforcing the power level coalition as a means of reducing the guilt and burden from the natural parent. Such an example would be:

---

[15]Alfred S. Friedman, et al. *Psychotherapy for the Whole Family*, New York, Springer Publishing Co., 1965, p. 308.

Identified Patient: I feel there is a great canyon between me and them. Everytime I try to jump over I fall about six feet short and start climbing up the wall.

Mother: Oh, what can I do to eliminate that?

Therapist: That does not seem too unusual. Your parent and stepparent were an established system before you returned. They had worked out many of their values and established many of their rules before you returned. They have opened their system to let you in. While rules are established within the system to accommodate you, it would be impossible for them to restructure their established system for you entirely.

The therapist may also want to identify which of the stages of Erickson's developmental stages the quasiadult has progressed to in development. Suggestions by the therapist may include experiences to assist the quasiadult through the developmental stages to the meet the current chronological age.

Another problem area may be in role expectations for the quasiadult in relation to the functioning of the system. This may take some compromising and/or bargaining to establish a mutually satisfying role pattern. The parents may be particularly anxious in this area. In one of the families seen, the mother related to the therapist her instructions by the psychiatrist to treat her son as a "disabled houseguest." It took several sessions discussing systems and some of the concepts to disspel the belief of harm that would come to them if they did not follow the psychiatrist's instructions.

The natural parent may feel threatened by unacceptable behavior of the quasiadult in the eyes of their marital partner and try very hard to be a "good parent." Such behavior on the part of the natural parent may hinder the growth and development of the quasiadult. The therapist can assist the family in understanding their own behavior, apparent goals, and end result. Such feelings on the part of the natural parent may result in the parent sending double messages to the quasiadult. An example would be:

Mother: I worried so about him after he got out of the service, I asked him to come and stay with us so he could rest and get well. If he weren't living here I wouldn't be so worried about him, but when he's here and I see him rotting away in that room and it tears me up.

These double messages are frequently implicit and places the recipient in an impossible situation. The sender of such messages needs to be made aware of the impossibility of the messages and motivated toward efforts to correct them. This involves the total system. Since the messages are sent unconsciously the receiver must say: "You've got me in an impossible situation" and further explain what was said.

Ackerman states that "it is possible to trace the individual's breakdown to a failure to find support within the family group for his personal need, for the solution of conflict, for the affirmation of a favored self-image and for the maintenance of necessary forms of defense against authority."[16] The therapist must look for a break in at least one of these areas. Since many of these activities are unconscious it is necessary for the therapist to identify the area to the family in such terminology that acceptance is possible by those contributing to the breakdown.

It may be necessary for the therapist to teach the family how to communicate what was intended to be communicated. It may also be necessary to teach the family how to clarify meanings before jumping to conclusions. Such an example would be:

Identified Patient: My Mother is so hard to understand. It is like there is a black veil over her to keep me from reading her.

Mother to Therapist: "Am I that hard to understand? Do you have trouble understanding me?

Therapist: No, I don't feel that way because I ask for explanations and interpretations to messages I fail to understand. It is not only the privilege of the family members to do the same but the obligation of them to clarify the meaning.

The therapist is obligated to set an example of behavior and communication patterns for role modeling within the system.

While new patterns of behavior may not be long established within the current system, the units of the system have brought with them faulty communication patterns, unresolved conflict, and unfulfilled needs if distress signals continue to be emitted within the new system. Because of the newness of the system and the patterns within the system that are in the process of being established, it may be easier for the therapist to teach new behavior and promote change.

[16]Nathan Ackerman, *The Psychodynamics of Family Life*, New York, Basic Books, Inc., 1958, p. 106.

BIBLIOGRAPHY

Ackerman Nathan. *The Psychodynamics of Family Life,* New York, Basic Books, Inc., 1958.

Bredemeier and Stephenson. *The Analysis of Social Systems,* New York, Holt, Rinehart and Winston, Inc., 1965.

Friedman, Alfreds, et al. *Psychotherapy for the Whole Family,* New York, Springer Publishing Co., 1965.

Haley, Jay. *Strategies of Psychotherapy,* New York, Grune and Stratton, 1963.

Horney, Karen. *Feminine Psychology,* New York, W. W. Norton and Co. Inc., 1967.

Lederer, William J. and Don D. Jackson. *The Mirages of Marriage,* New York, W. W. Norton and Co., Inc., 1968.

McCandless, Boyd R. *Adolescent Behavior and Development,* Hindsdale, Ill., The Dryden Press, Inc., 1970.

Satir, Virginia. *Conjoint Family Therapy,* Palo Alto, Calif., Science and Behavior Books, Inc., 1967.

Part III
COVERT COMMUNICATION MODES

9.

Sham in a Family

Jeannine Dunwell

To some degree, all persons in family systems use sham or masking. Henry supports this proposition and states, "The child makes sham a natural part of life by seeing parents practice it and then turns the tables on them.[1]

A problem arises from the reciprocating effect the use of masking behavior by family members has within the family system. The consequences of this behavior and a description of the interventions of the therapist to effect change in the system are presented to acquaint the reader with the ever-widening outcomes of masking and unmasking. This selection illustrates how one family used sham with reciprocating effects that resulted in a reversal of roles for parents and children.

A review of the literature and clinical examples of behaviors and interventions are included. Results of the interventions with recommendations for modifications of interventions are described. Names of family members have been changed to insure anonymity.

OVERVIEW AND FOCUS

As each family member attempted to use sham to maintain a valued role within the system, the therapist observed resulting miscommunication of messages in this family system.

Lederer and Jackson describe the use of sham by the marital dyad to put up a front that "all is well with the marriage and family;" the result is emotionally sick children. They state that interventions by the therapist

[1]Jules Henry, "The Anatomy of Sham," *Pathways to Madness*, Part II, New York, Random House, 1971, p. 107.

that serve to facilitate communication within the system can effect an unmasking that will benefit all relationships with the system.[2]

To make this concept more functional, the following operational definition is stated:

"Reciprocating Shamasking"

1. Stated or idealized expectations of family members do not match underlying real expectations.

2. This mismatch is covert and denied.

3. Mutual fear of unmasking occurs in all family members.

4. Parents and children use this as threat.

5. The reciprocating effect of masking behavior is the creation of a greater need for masking by the other persons in the system.

The therapist has chosen to focus upon the miscommunications within the system caused when expectations stated do not match the underlying message and the sham is compounded by covert behavior.

REVIEW OF THE LITERATURE

Henry states that the more vulnerable one feels, the more likely one is to conceal feelings and erect a facade. He further states that children become high tension wires bearing the electricity of parental deception.[3]

Henry defines sham as a combination of concealment and pretense. He illustrates this by referring to two concentric circles: One is "The Inner Circle," which refers to beliefs held about the self and shared with intimate friends or family. Here, he says, is the ideal circle of truth where there can be no concealment. The other area, "The Outer Circle," refers to relationships with the broader system, such as relatives, organizations, or occupational associates. Here, he states, concealment and pretense are the best policy because the truth would be sheer stupidity. He says that concealment is a social obligation in getting along in the outer world, but this gives rise to problems when "The Inner Circle" requires concealment and a person reveals truth in "The Outer Circle."[4]

The family described here used sham in *both* the inner and outer circles, requiring pretense upon pretense to maintain the system.

The concept of reciprocating effect of behaviors in a family system is documented by Branch, who describes the family as a conveyor belt for

---

[2]William J. Lederer and Don D. Jackson, *Mirages of Marriage,* New York, W. W. Norton & Co., Inc., 1968, pp. 153-160.

[3]Henry, *op. cit.,* p. 101.

[4]*Ibid.,* pp. 99-102.

anxiety and conflict with all members affecting the mental health of other members within the system. He states that even minor emotional deviations of one member within the family can have undeniable repercussions, often present in deviant behavior and distorted interpersonal relationships. The member who appears most disturbed may actually not be the cause of the real trouble but may be "acting out" in response to behaviors of other members in the system.[5] This concept is important to remember as the clinical data are explored.

Observing techniques used by couples who are fearful of having the marriage relationship explored, Framo concluded that many parents use problems of the children as dilatory tactics to ward off exploration.[6] This may be viewed as another form of masking to avoid focusing on unmet expectations of the marital dyad.

The importance of communication and miscommunication in the relationships of family members is stressed by Satir, who states that communication, both verbal and nonverbal, can indicate the quality of the relationships. Unclear communications mean that it is impossible for members in the system to differentiate and relate to persons and objects within the system. *Meta*communication is defined as a comment on the literal message as well as the nature of the relationship between the persons involved. It conveys the sender's attitude about the message he sends. Incongruent messages are two or more messages sent at different levels that contradict each other. This places a burden on the receiver if he is to find out what is really being said. Incongruence leads to stalemating, and clear congruent communication leads to growth in the learning process and, hence, in the quality of interpersonal relations.[7] This explanation of the effect of incongruence seems to bear a direct relationship to maintenance of sham or the clarification of messages on all levels that would contribute to unmasking.

Spiegel describes role dislocation as a process of avoiding conflicts in a role system by rearranging the role partner's position relative to each other or the trade-off of roles as a way to limit conflict without facing the issues involved in role discrepancy.[8] This description indicates that role dislocation also contributes to the sham.

[5]C. H. Hardin Branch, *Aspects of Anxiety,* Philadelphia, J. B. Lippincott Co., 1965, pp. 117-127.

[6]James L. Framo, "Rationale and Techniques of Intensive Family Therapy," *Intensive Family Therapy,* Ivan Bozormenyi-Nagy and James L. Framo, eds., New York, Harper & Row, 1965, p. 188.

[7]Virginia Satir, *Conjoint Family Therapy,* Palo Alto, Science and Behavior Books, Inc., 1967, pp. 75-90.

[8]John Spiegel, *Transactions, The Interplay Between Individual, Family and Society,* New York, Science House, Inc., 1971.

CLINICAL DATA

The Smith family consisted of a mother, age 39, a father, age 45, a daughter, Jane, age 16, and a son, Bill, age 14.

After observing the use of sham by all members in this family system, it was hypothesized by the therapist that a process of the children parenting or punishing the parents was occurring. The fact that both children were adopted suggested that these parents might be more vulnerable than other parents in similar situations because of fear of loss of love of the children. This factor would seem to contribute to the perpetuation of the "protection" of the sham.

Sham was displayed by family members both verbally and nonverbally. In the beginning sessions, Mr. S. would sit very straight in his chair with arms (and sometimes legs) crossed. He also verbalized that he was a good provider of material things for his family. He said his wife fulfilled all his expectations by cooking, keeping the house neat, and going on trips with him. Mrs. S. concurred with Mr. S. in that he fulfilled her expectations in his provider role and she was happy meeting his expectations of her as cook and housekeeper.

The mixed messages then began to flow:

Mr. S.: Like I always tell my kids, you should go right on to college, because if you don't, you will find you soon have obligations of a house, a family, bills . . . . I wanted to go on to college.

This statement was made just after he had stated how happy he was in his job.

Mrs. S.: I can't get involved with Jane's problems outside the home because I just fall apart and can't cope. My husband always goes.

Further data revealed that she had gone with Jane to the probation officer and on occasion went to pick up Jane when she was stranded and the father refused to go. These two examples seem to illustrate a case of "Your lips tell me 'no, no' but there's 'yes, yes' in your eyes."

Messages from parents to children were not clear. Literal statement and intent were not congruent. For example:

*Mr. S.:*You know you are supposed to be in by eleven o'clock.

J: But you've said if I call to let you know where I am, I might stay later.

Mr. S.: Well, yes, but not always.

The children observed the use of the "white lie" by parents and used it effectively to gain what they wanted. Disapproval of this practice was stated by parents, followed by Mr. S. saying, "Well, one time is O.K.; nobody's perfect."

There was much miscommunication in the family over expectations of members to fulfill responsibilities that went unmet. These are described as *ad hoc* rules and jobs that are done "for" the parents.

Mrs. S.: The children are expected to keep their rooms clean, but if they don't I'll go in and clean them after so long.

Mr. S.: Well, they usually clean them if they're asked.

This come back through the children's communication when they said, "I usually do it — about one-fourth the time." The same ratio was stated about emptying the dishwasher and other jobs.

The threat of unmasking was shown when Bill, teasingly, told his parents he was going to tell something they didn't know and proceeded to confess breaking of a family rule in the past. This elicited a mixed response from parents, a look of anxiety before he stated it, and a rationalization of his behavior after the confession.

Parenting behavior in the role reversal took on different forms for Bill and Jane. Bill performed readily rewardable behaviors such as arranging an anniversary party for the parents, not allowing Jane to help, and continued to hear parents praise him. Jane "punished" the parents by behaviors that embarrassed them in front of friends. She smoked pot, wore sloppy jeans, "talked back to teachers," had been arrested for possession of marijuana, and moved out to live with her boyfriend for one week. The strongest indication that she used her behavior to punish the parents was illustrated by the following:

I guess I wanted revenge when I started to rebel, because they had been so strict with me. Now they're much more lenient with Bill. It's not fair.

The masking behavior used by the parents and children jointly was evident when Jane would say, "I usually do" or "sometimes do" when speaking of expectations of the parents concerning being in on time. Then the parents would say, "She's good about calling when she's going to be late — usually." Excuses were given for behavior, thus making the message unclear about expectations. The excuses and rationalization by the parents, which masked the stating of what happened, resulted in masking statements from the children to perpetuate the myth that "what happened in this family really wasn't so painful." Similarly, masking statements made by the children brought masking responses from the parents. This was seen as reciprocating behavior.

Resistance to unmasking was seen in all members, but illustrated best by Jane's statement:

I just don't see any problems here. When did this family get the idea there was a big problem.

STRATEGIES FOR INTERVENTION

Family therapy that involves the therapist and the family in interaction in the home of the family was chosen as the mode of treatment for this family because this therapy mode focuses on the extant systems network with the therapist working to maintain patterns of interaction that are judged to promote growth while working to promote change in patterns that restrict growth.[9] One pattern of interaction that the therapist observed as restrictive to growth — the use of sham and sending of mixed messages — was the focus for interventions described here.

The therapist chose to intervene at this point in the process because of the reciprocating use of sham. It was thought that clarification of what was said and what was, in fact, expected would decrease the need for the family to use sham and would effect a change in the reciprocating pattern.

In describing interventions for dealing with covert communication, Satir states:

When asking and accusing become this hidden, any third party looking on becomes confused and asks, "Who wants what from whom?"

a. A child in the family can become confused.

b. A therapist can become confused unless he sees to it that wishes and accusations get clearly labeled as coming from someone and going toward someone.[10]

Satir's rationale for unmasking is that it serves to help family members to say what they see, think, and feel, and to bring disagreements out in the open. She says,

I especially want mates to see where they have been giving conflicting messages to their children as well as each other. Marital communication sets the standard for parental communication and for all communication between family members.[11]

Clarification was sought by the therapist by repeatedly asking questions to clarify the meanings of terms used by family members with insistence that they be stated behaviorally.

Mr. S.: My wife loses her temper.

T: What does she do?

Mr. S.: She yells at the kids, slams doors and bangs cupboard doors.

T: For how long?

Mr. S.: Thirty minutes to an hour.

---

[9]Grayce Sills, lecture notes, August 4, 1972. University of New Mexico, Psychiatric Nursing Workshop.
[10]Satir, *op. cit.*, p. 10.
[11]*Ibid.*, p. 11.

The following dialogues describe some of Satir's strategies for intervention with examples of their use in this family system:

Satir: *Additional statements are made by the therapist to point out discrepancies in messages.*[12]

J.: Mother doesn't want me to smoke pot in the house because it bothers her sinuses.

T.: Then you are saying it's O.K. to smoke it outside where your sinuses aren't?

Mrs. S.: Well, no, I don't want her to smoke it at all, but I've told her it bothers my sinuses if she smokes it in here. But *I don't want her to smoke it at all.*

J.: Dad doesn't feel the same. He doesn't fear it because he's read research in "Playboy" so he doesn't totally disapprove.

T.: Is that what you said?

Mr. S.: No, I disapprove, too, because it is harmful and illegal.

T.: There seems to have been a mixed message in what was said and heard. Do you now hear your Mom and Dad saying the same thing?

Satir: *The therapist educates for discrepancies in messages about accountability. When he deals with acting out of children he doesn't turn to parents, he asks the child "How come?" He reminds the child that he has a choice about his behavior. He isn't a victim. He can influence his environment.*[13]

T.: You moved out of the house and lived with your boyfriend, but you are living here at home now. How did you make that decision?

J.: I don't know. I liked living in both places.

T.: But one can't live in two places at once. You made the choice to live here. What is it you like here?

J.: Well, the convenience, the color T.V., no dogs running through the house, a cleaner house, a vacuum cleaner, iron, and dishwasher.

Satir: *The therapist spells out "double level" messages.*[14]

Mrs. S.: Well the kids know they are to clean their rooms.

T.: How does that go?

Mrs. S.: Well, if they don't, I tell them three or four times, then I get mad and either they do it or I clean it. They do it about one out of four times.

[12]*Ibid.*, p. 70.
[13]*Ibid.*, p. 173.
[14]*Ibid.*, p. 176.

T.: You are saying to them that what is expected of them is that about one-fourth the time they will clean their rooms, but if they don't, you will.

Another intervention, used as a modification of one suggested by Satir, was decreasing threat by reducing the need for defenses by using humor. The therapist exaggerated discrepancies in statements which served to decrease tension and point out the discrepancy.[15]

J.: Requirements? There aren't any requirements at my school.

T.: What is it you've got going here in A_____? Some kind of magical school where nobody has to do anything?

J.: Well, there *are* some requirements, like grades and homework.

One written assignment, suggested by Smoyak, was used to clarify discrepancies in stated expectations of family members for each other.[16] Each member was asked to write five times in each labeled square. This instrument was expanded to include squares for each member to make statements about each other member.

a. Things about me I like and don't want to change:	b. Things about spouse I like and don't want to change:
1.	1.
2.	2.
3.	3.
4.	4.
5.	5.

c. Things about me I don't like and am willing to change:	d. Things about spouse I don't like and want him or her to change:
1.	1.
2.	2.
3.	3.
4.	4.
5.	5.

---

[15]*Ibid.*, p. 168.

[16]Shirley Smoyak, lecture notes, July 28, 1972, University of New Mexico, Psychiatric Nursing Workshop.

The instrument proved not only to be an excellent strategy for pointing out discrepancies and for members to learn new things about each other but was also a catalyst used to unmask and interact issues, without exhibiting a need for the mask.

The results of the interventions described indicated this family was capable of producing change in the masking behavior by using less verbal and nonverbal incongruent behavior. The father no longer sat with arms and legs crossed, and the mother no longer "dressed up" for the therapy sessions. They had learned to look at some discrepancies and to try to define terms they used.

In continued work with this family on the problems of reciprocating sham, it was the recommendation of the therapist to continue to "pin them down" in clarifying messages, to assist them in finding some meaningful rewards for desired behavior of system members — especially rewards that were not material — and to work to establish an increasing number of *quid pro quos*. It was the opinion of the therapist that it would have been more effective to move in quicker with more force in approach because the therapist underestimated the strength of the resistance to change in the use of sham.

SUMMARY

The use of sham, with its reciprocating consequences, was demonstrated by this family system. The concept of reciprocating effect is a most useful one for the therapist when working with the family system; as in this situation, the effect of change is also reciprocating. One cannot drop the mask a little without having an effect on the system. However, the therapist should not underestimate the resistance to unmasking and giving up of the protective sham. It spells hard work for the therapist and hard work for the family.

BIBLIOGRAPHY

Branch, C. H. Hardin. *Aspects of Anxiety,* Philadelphia, J. B. Lippincott Co., 1965.

Framo, James L. "Rationale and Techniques of Intensive Family Therapy," *Intensive Family Therapy,* Ivan Bozormenyi-Nagy and James L. Framo, eds., New York, Harper & Row, 1965.

Henry, Jules. "The Anatomy of Sham," *Pathways to Madness,* Part II, New York, Random House, 1965.

Lederer, William J. and Don D. Jackson. *Mirages of Marriage,* New York, W. W. Norton & Co., Inc., 1968.

Satir, Virginia. *Conjoint Family Therapy.* Palo Alto, Science and Behavior Books, Inc., 1967.

Sills, Grayce. Lecture notes, August 4, 1972, University of New Mexico, Psychiatric Nursing Workshop.

Spiegel, John. *Transactions, The Interplay Between Individual, Family and Society,* New York, Science House, Inc., 1971.

Smoyak, Shirley. Lecture notes, July 28, 1972, University of New Mexico, Psychiatric Nursing Workshop.

10.

Family Myths

Helen Brandt Battiste

The concept of "family myth" is discussed here as one dynamic factor in families who have developed rigidity of their mutual roles and a limited variety of interactional patterns. The process of myth making as a phenomenon of human beings in groups is presented to provide some insights into family myth making.

When operationally defined, the concept of family myths has some direct implications for development of clinical guidelines.

I. FAMILIES

Many families seen in family therapy seem, to the therapist, to have interactional patterns within their systems that are strikingly without variety. For example, in some families, after one session of family therapy, the therapist may feel that he could predict accurately who will say what, who will do what, who will tell who what to do and how, how decisions will be managed and so on.

These families seem to have a limited repertoire for dealing with life. But this is not to say that they disintegrate in crises. On the contrary, their narrow range of ways to react seems to have provided the necessary closeness and stability to hold the family together.

There have been many terms to describe various phenomena noted about the rigid roles and fixed interactional patterns in families. Lidz and Fleck[1] used the concept of "schism and skew," and Wynne,[2] et. al., used

[1]T. Lidz, A. Cornelison, S. Fleck, and D. Terry. "The Intrafamilial Environment of the Schizophrenic Patient: II. Marital Schism and Skew," *American Journal of Psychiatry*, 1957, *114*:241–248.

[2]L. Wynne, I. Ryhoff, J. Day, and S. Hirsh, "Pseudomutuality in the Family Relations of Schizophrenics," *Psychiatry*, 1958, *21*:205–220.

the concept of "pseudomutuality" (previously called the "rubber fence"). Ackerman[3] talked of "interlocking pathology" and Bowen[4] of "undifferentiated ego mass." Recently Pittman and Flomenhaft[5] wrote of "Doll's House Marriages," drawing parallels with the relationships of characters in Ibsen's play. Other terms refer to these families' interactional systems as "binding," "stuck togeher," and "interlocking."

When their characteristics are described, and their dynamics explored, these families seem to operate on the principle that *one act equals one response.* An event occurs, and a predictable pattern of response is automatically set in motion. However compromising to the family system, however restricting to the individuals in the family, however strange to those outside the family or the culture, however "pathological" to the therapist — these rigid and limited responses by the family have served to hold the family together.

How then do these families get into family therapy? It seems that this is when some new or unpredicted event occurs for which there is no rehearsed reaction. Some of the events might be loss or threat of loss of a family member, physical illnesses, geographical moves, or movement from one socioeconomic level to another, for example. One or more family members, influenced by factors outside the family such as school, may begin to question the family systems. (Why do we have to do things this way?) One or more members may have symptoms of emotional illness or deviant social behavior. An outside agency, such as a school, might insist that there is "pathology" in a member.

Whatever the circumstances that bring these families to treatment, the therapist does not assume that since the usual ways of interacting in the family system are not working, the family is anxious to try new alternatives. The old ways are sometimes painful, but at least it's pain they know about. New ways are frightening because the family lacks a predictive frame.

Ferreira[6] suggests that many families seek psychiatric assistance in order not to change, that is, as part of the effort to maintain the status quo of the family. Particularly where there is an identified "patient" or a "troublemaker" of some sort in the family constellation, the spoken or unspoken reason for seeking or accepting outside help is so that person can be "straightened up" and things will be all right with the family again.

[3]N. Ackerman, "Interlocking Pathology in Family Relationships," *Changing Concepts in Psychoanalytical Medicine,* Sandn Rado and G. E. Daniels, eds., New York, Grune and Stratton, 1956.

[4]Murray Bowen, "The Use of Family Theory in Clinical Practice," *Comprehensive Psychiatry,* Vol. 7, 1966, pp. 345–374.

[5]Frank S. Pittman, III, and Kalman Flomenhaft, "Treating the Doll's House Marriage," *Family Process, 9,* June 1970, pp. 143–155.

[6]Antonio Ferreira, "Family Myths," *Psychiatric Research Reports 20,* 1966, p. 88.

It is here that the therapist ponders, "how did this family get this way?" "And how can I intervene in this system to help make it more functional for all members?"

II. MYTHS

Myths have been a part of man's culture from earliest times. They were tales and legends passed from one generation to another, telling of supernatural feats, superiority over enemies, and over evil forces. They tell where people came from, what kind of people they were, and how they survived. They explain natural phenomena, thus giving some clues that people could use to avoid bad outcomes for themselves.

Myth[7] "has come into popular usage to mean any invented story. In sociology and anthropology, however, a myth is a collective belief that is built up in response to the wishes of the group, instead of a rational analysis of the situation to which it pertains."

That myths have this relationship to the wishes of groups would explain why myths have persisted in man's history. Consider the myth, "My nation (tribe, race, group) is morally superior to any other." This belief seems necessary to the survival of any such groups. How else can individuals in nations, tribes, races, and other groups justify their aggressive, hostile, or provocative actions toward other groups?

Individuals often have private doubts and questions about national, racial, and group myths but to question them openly has its hazards. The individual may experience considerable anxiety if he no longer holds the myths to be true since the realities and facts of living may be complicated and hard to accept. In addition, other group members are likely to react with anger toward someone who openly challenges the myths, even though they as individuals may have private doubts.

Gregory Rochlin[8] speaks of myths as functioning for groups of people much as wish-fulfilling fantasies function for individuals:

The motives for myth-making and the function of myths are in such close harmony that it would be artificial to attempt a sharp separation. The human psychological condition regularly reveals in its conflicts that throughout life uncertainty remains, risk exists, and unpredictability in human relationships and events persists. These facts of life are learned remarkably early. Fantasy formation and its communal form, myth-making, are best understood as functions aimed at the needs of wish

---

[7]Bergen Evans and C. Evans, *Dictionary of Contemporary American Usage,* New York, Random House, 1957.

[8]Gregory Rochlin, *Griefs and Discontents, the Forces of Change,* Boston, Little, Brown and Company, 1965, pp. 135.

fulfillment. The content of myths draws from wishes often expressed as fantasies. Some of the sources may be unconscious. The motive for myth-making, in part, is a form of the need of a defense against the limitations that living imposes.

He also states that myths have one basic principle: they abolish or suspend the laws of reality. Myths will show that limitations may be transcended and that there are no bounds.

Obviously groups *do* deal directly with many of these facts of life that seem contrary to their wishes and expectations of life. These confrontations between wishes and reality lead to greater flexibility in how the groups operate. When anxiety is too great, however, myth making rather than confrontations frequently occur.

It follows that the more myths a group has, the less flexibility it has. The rules about who in the group does what, when, how, and under what conditions can be justified readily by referring to the myths. There is no need to examine situations and to try to figure out the best ways to react. There are rules that can't be questioned because they are based on the myths, so that's the way it has to be.

For example let us say that a group has a myth, "only males over 57½ years of age have the wisdom to be our leaders." Rules and laws are then made that exclude women and all males under 57½ years. The process of selection is less complicated and more routinized. The group functions with little or no anxiety and stress if all believe the myth.

Then a calamity strikes all males over 57½ years old. This group now becomes immobilized because it has developed no alternative criteria for selecting leaders. It has followed one pattern (it needed only one pattern since it was based on the myth that said that they already knew who were the best leaders). Although this example is obviously simplistic and improbable, it serves to highlight the dysfunctionality of myths.

III. FAMILY MYTH

Ferreira[9] defines the concept of family myth as "a series of fairly well integrated beliefs shared by all family members, concerning each other and their mutual position in the family life, beliefs that go unchallenged by everyone involved, in spite of the reality distortions they may conspiciously imply." He notes that these beliefs are different from the "front" or social facade that the family as a group attempts to present to outsiders. The myths are part of the inner image of the group.

[9]A. J. Ferreira, "Family Myth and Homeostasis," *Arch. Gen. Psychiatry*, 9, 1963, pp. 457–463.

Examples of families beliefs about itself are, "Mother needs us to take care of her"; "We all like to do things together"; "We stay married only because of the children"; "Father is the strong one"; "We drive mother in the car; she's too nervous"; "We all share the household chores"; "We're a happy family". When these inner images a family has of itself seem to not ring true to the outside observer, but when the family clings tenaciously to them, one is probably on the track of a family myth.

An important distinction between the concept of family myth and the kinds of reality distortions that are a part of most families must be made. For instance, a family may distort reality when recalling how much fun it was "the time they were stuck in the mud and had to sleep in the car." But they are willing to admit that really it wasn't so much fun. They were frightened, they couldn't sleep, etc. Furthermore, these kinds of stories are seldom used to justify how the family functions as it does in the present. Ferreira speculates that most real family myths have their origin in the early days of the family, when formulas for "togetherness" are being actively sought, and the future of the relationship seems uncertain. He sees the function of family myths then as a "homeostatic" one — meaning that it provides the basis for governor reactions. Furthermore, it promotes closeness. "But like any homeostatic mechanism, it tends to maintain and even to increase the level of organization in the family by establishing patterns that perpetuate themselves with circularity and self correction."[10]

This increase in the level of organization, and development of circular patterns — based on a myth — does seem to preserve the family. What it does not promote is the feeling of confidence and growth that comes from having dealt with life in a non-stereotypic way, experienced shared disappointments, tried out alternatives, and mastered situations by new solutions.

Family myth may be operationalized this way:

1. Family members bring into the family expectations and wishes that are culturally, socially, and biologically determined.

2. When family systems encounter the realities of family living, many expectations are not met.

3. The family system does not confront the reality that threatens its expectations, but instead preserves its status quo by denying reality.

4. Family develops beliefs that state that the family system is what they would like it to be (i.e., that expectations are being met).

5. These beliefs are reinforced and continue to be held collectively and

[10]Ibid., p. 60.

are supported by the family as if they were ultimate truth and beyond challenge because:

a. The beliefs determine how family members initiate, maintain, and justify their mutual roles and interactional patterns.

b. They promote automatic agreement and formation of rituals, which are stabilizing, reassuring, and promote closeness.

c. They provide satisfaction for the family, that its beliefs about itself are reality.

A clinical application of the concept of family myth is illustrated by the Leit family. This family sought help from a child guidance clinic, because of their concern with their 14-year-old son's behavior. They saw him as irresponsible, stubborn, disobedient, and a candidate for the juvenile detention home.

From the first session, the therapist noted that Mr. and Mrs. L. had quite different approaches to life. He experienced life in a cognitive way, she in an emotional way. And yet when they were asked to describe how they got their ideas of what a family should be like, Mrs. L. emphatically stated that fortunately for them, their backgrounds were alike, "We are both French Canadian Catholics from the Northeast."

She repeated this theme several times in following sessions. She explained that while she realized her children were growing up in the Southwest, she and her husband still preserved intact their own values and standards of conduct and tried to pass them on to their children.

During the first session, the therapist gave both husband and wife an assignment, in order to give them some idea of their "differentness." Mr. L. was asked to "feel one feeling this week and come to the next session ready to describe it," Mrs. L. was asked to "think one thought and report on that." Both had considerable difficulty in carrying out these tasks, Mr. L. remarking, "Its imposible for me to have a feeling, unless I think about it first." Both, however, made repented statements about their "alikeness." The strategy was to get them to acknowledge difference between them, so that they could move toward acknowledging and allowing differences in their son.

During following sessions of course, many instances of the husband and wife's "differentness" came to light with no attempt on the part of the therapist to "unmask" or attack the myth that they were alike, but merely to comment on what is observed. For example, (following discussion of very different reactions on the part of he and his wife, to one child's behavior):

Therapist: How is it that things that bother Mrs. Leit don't bother you?

Mr. L.: Chemicals.

Therapist: How's that? Did you say chemicals?

Mr. L.: The time of the month, you know (smiling).

Therapist: Is that right!

He was able to acknowledge biological difference much more readily than ideological difference.

In a discussion of how they met and married, it becomes apparent that the expectations of each were not met in the early marriage situation. Mrs. L., who was attracted to her husband because he was a "snob," talked bitterly of working to support him while he was unemployed and a student. Mr. L. described his wife as the prominent girl on campus, active, busy, a cheerleader. He emphasized that she was quite different then and laughingly said he had thought of her as a "fast woman."

The therapist's question to Mrs. L., "Now how did a staunch French Canadian Catholic from the Northeast get to be a 'fast woman'?" was answered by Mrs. L., "Oh, he thought I was 'fast' because I was in so many activities and always doing things."

Later in that session the following interaction took place:

Mrs. L.: As I've said, we're very compatible.

Therapist: How are you compatible?

Mr. L. to Mrs. L.: How are we compatible?

Mrs. L.: We're alike.

Therapist: How are you alike?

Mrs. L.: Well, because we come from the same backgrounds. You remember, I told you we were French Canadian Catholics. Have you read *Evangeline?*

Therapist to Mrs. L.: I do remember you told me you were a purebred.

Mr. L.: I'm a mongrel.

Therapist: What?

Mr. L.: "I'm a mongrel and it doesn't both me.

Therapist to Mrs. L.: It's important for you to be alike.

Mr. L.: Well, it's important for her to be French —

Therapist: I said, its important for her to be alike.

This beginning acceptance of "differentness," which could be called the doing away of the myth, was not accomplished as an end in itself. It provided a chance for them to understand how myth defense patterns developed early in the family, which avoided the discomfort of the anxiety of reconciling differences. Their interactions and the mutual roles assumed fell into a stereotypic mythical program. The myth that they were alike made negotiations seem unnecessary, and so rules, contracts, and agreements between husband and wife about who has the right to do what, to whom, and under what conditions "just seemed to happen." Indeed, this family, like many others, did not really notice that they had any contracts and agreements between themselves.

In therapy, this family became more aware of alternative patterns of interaction. Who controls what part of the family life *can* be negotiated, for example, with the adolescents only after the solidarity myth is dispelled. The myth of "alikeness" was challenged by the son, who was responding to the need for developing autonomy. Mr. Leit, on the other hand, thought of his son as so "irresponsible" that he, the father, should retain control over all aspects of his son's life with the exception of his eating, drinking, breathing, and excretory functions. When "alikeness" is dispelled as a myth, all have more freedom to move and grow.

The clinical application of the concept of family myth are summarized in this way:

1. The therapist takes note of the items that the family states are true about itself but that don't "ring true."

2. The therapist does attempt to validate these clues by getting further data from the family. He also tries to match his clues to what he observes of the patterns for how the family functions as a system.

3. The therapist avoids attacking these myths since it is likely that the family will react with anger. It is also important to remember that the family will give clues about what myths they are ready to question and which not.

4. He focuses the family back to its beginnings, on the theory that myths are ways to avoid the pain of unmet expectations, especially in beginning relationships. Family may reveal new information about themselves as individuals and what their expectations and wishes were.

5. Therapist moves the family back to the present and begins to encourage negotiations among family members in areas where myths operated previously. The family is encouraged to work out their roles and interactional patterns on the basis of "this is what I want (expect, wish, need). I will give up something for you, if I can get this."

BIBLIOGRAPHY

Ackerman, N. "Interlocking Pathology in Family Relationships," *Changing Concepts in Psychoanalytical Medicine,* Sandn Rado and G. E. Daniels, eds., New York, Grune and Stratton, 1956.

Bowen, Murray. "The Use of Family Theory in Clinical Practice, *Comprehensive Psychiatry,* Vol. 7, 1966, pp. 345–374.

Evans, Bergen and C. Evans. *Dictionary of Contemporary American Usage,* New York, Random House, 1957.

Ferreira, Antonio. "Family Myths:, *Psychiatric Research Reports, 20,* 1966, pp. 85–90.

Ferreira, A. J. "Family Myth and Homeostatis," *Arch. Gen. Psychiatry, 9,* 1963, pp. 457–463.

Friedman et al. *Psychotherapy for the Whole Family,* New York, Springer Publishing Company, Inc., 1965.

Lederer, William J. and Don D. Jackson. *The Mirages of Marriage,* New York, W. W. Norton & Co., Inc., 1968.

Lidz, T., A. Cornelison, S. Fleck, and D. Terry. "The Intrafamilial Environment of the Schizophrenic Patient: II. Marital Schism and Skew," *American Journal of Psychiatry,* 1957, *114*:241–248.

Pittman, Frank S. III and Kalman Flomenhaft. "Treating the Doll's House Marriage," *Family Process,* Vol. 9, June 1970, pp. 143–155.

Rochlin, Gregory. *Griefs and Discontents, the Forces of Change,* Boston: Little, Brown and Company, 1965.

Smoyak, Shirley A. "Threat: A Recurring Family Dynamic," *Perspectives in Psychiatric Care,* Vol. VII, 1969, pp. 267–274.

Speigel, Rose. "Specific Problems of Communication in Psychiatric Conditions," *American Handbook of Psychiatry,* Vol. I, pp. 909–949.

Wynne, L., I. Ryhoff, J. Day, and S. Hirsch. "Pseudomutuality in the Family Relations of Schizophrenics," *Psychiatry,* 1958, *21*:205–220.

11.

Solidarity Versus Pseudomutuality

Ida Silver

As a social system, the family consists of persons who relate to each other in varying modes. The transactions that exist within the family structure will determine the difference between healthy relationships as opposed to pathological functioning.

"The systems concept postulates that there is a constant action-interaction between associated things. The closer the association, the more obvious is the action-reaction. If an influence upsets the balance between associated entities, then a compensatory factor is provided by the system to regain balance."[1]

In this selection, the issue of a pathological pattern is defined, described, and discussed in order to demonstrate how a pathological system of interaction within a family is a causative factor in schizophrenia. The type of relationship is pseudomutuality. Wynne calls it "a type of relatedness in which there is a preoccupation of family members with a fitting together into formal roles at the expense of individual identity."[2]

The opposite of pseudomutuality is solidarity. Close relationships between members over a long period of time, commitment and feelings of warmth and mutuality, result in solidarity. Feelings of solidarity are very important in dealing with individual tensions and personality problems.[3]

Solidarity is defined as a "preponderance of favorable affects over hostile affects, and a similar balance of moral respect over moral con-

[1]William J. Lederer and Don D. Jackson, *The Mirages of Marriage*, New York, W. W. Norton & Co., 1968, p. 88.

[2]Gerald H. Zuk and David Rubinstein, "A Review of Concepts in the Study and Treatment of Families of Schizophrenics," *Intensive Family Therapy*, New York, Harper & Row 1965, p. 13.

[3]Norman W. Bell and Ezra F. Vogel, "Toward a Framework for Functional Analysis of Family Behavior," *The Family*, New York, The Free Press, 1968, p. 25.

demnation among the participants of the system."[4] The family as a social system is responsible for transmitting the social heritage to the new generation. This facilitates its absorption into the larger society as the bearer of a particular culture. In socializing the child, the parents are free to impose sanctions as a restraint toward deviance. They also reward him for the internalization of states of mind valued in the culture.

Family solidarity is maintained by ritual activities, vacation experiences, sexual relationships, and various expressions of affection. If the solidarity of a family is threatened by an outside source, the members mobilize their resources to preserve the ties. When members decide to separate from the family (and this is accomplished only after attempts by the other members to prevent this disruption) solidarity is disbanded. The problem that needs to be solved is how much solidarity versus autonomy for individual members will be allowed in the family?

In an ever-changing society, there are sources of strain operating against the attainment of family solidarity. On the one hand, the child is prepared for his role as a member of the larger community and, on the other hand, he is told to develop strong family ties. Another aspect of strain is caused by the progressive secularization of the culture. Parental control and traditionalism are being challenged. More emphasis is exerted toward a rational justification of beliefs and practices.

Boys, especially, are influenced by the peer society, with different values from those inculcated in the home. Values learned in the home are repudiated. In present society there exists a personal striving for material and prestige goals. Power, enjoyment, and freedom from anxiety are more significant for the individual than Christian values.

When the parents fail in their attempts to socialize the child because of his participation in the peer group (from whom he has adopted deviant practices), the reason for failure is attributed to outside forces. Tensions are reduced and conflict is averted because the child is considered beyond family control. Consequently, if the family is not to blame, intervention is futile.

Cousins, in "The Failure of Solidarity," offers three patterns of responsive intervention, which are made by family members in coping with the problem of the child's solidarity relationship to his family.[5]

1. Continuity. The parent attempts to force the normative goals of socialization upon the child by imposing sanctions or withdrawing the child from the asocial situation.

[4]Albert N. Cousins, "The Failure of Solidarity," *The Family*, New York, The Free Press, 1960, p. 403.
[5]Ibid., pp. 408–413.

2. Canalization. The parent directs the activities of the child into situations where his role as a member of a kinship group will come into play. School activities, church, and scouting fall into this group.

3. Discontinuity. The parent does not regard the cultural modes of socialization as goals that he himself has determined. He refrains from discussing controversial topics; he does not tell the child that something is good or bad, right or wrong.

It is interesting to perceive the adjustments made by the family in the society and, at the same time, their efforts to preserve solidarity. Perhaps, this can be attributed to the existence of true mutuality. In true mutuality the family members are able to experience personal identity and separateness. However, in pseudomutuality, divergence is forbidden. It is perceived as leading to a disruption of the relationship.

Within the family used for illustration here, where one member was schizophrenic, there was a limited number of fixed roles. The family consists of a father, mother and 28-year-old son, who is living at home, awaiting discharge from the service because of "paranoia" and a "persecution complex." Two older siblings are living in different parts of the country. A younger brother is presently in the military service. Family members may shift in these roles or compete for more desirable roles. A pseudomutual structure is typified by a paucity of possible roles, that is, there is a limited variety of available role positions or styles. It is not clear in this family whether the son is the social companion of the mother or the little boy needing care.

The pseudomutual structure is supported by myths and ideologies about the family. Children are rewarded when they behave with uniformity and punished for independent behavior. There is a mutual disregard for each other's autonomous needs.

During the course of a therapy session, the mother interrupts her son and interprets the father's statements. She presumes to know what the other members are feeling. For instance,

Mother: I felt hurt for him (son). I know how he was feeling.

Nurse: How did you know that?

Mother: I don't know. I think when you're close to a person . . .

Son: By my actions . . .

Mother: (interrupts) I don't know how he feels about her (girlfriend). But I felt bad for him. He had planned this meeting.

(Note the son, presumably the victim, participating in the same pattern.)
The following will again illustrate a disregard for autonomous otherness:

Nurse: What do you want for your son?

Mother: Happiness.

Nurse: Happiness means different things to different people . . .

Mother: I want Steve to do what he wants to do. Whatever is best for him. He can do anything.

Nurse: Anything is a broad term.

Mother: If he wants to go to school or go to work. He can do that. He is more than welcome here. Being home has helped him a lot.

The nurse intervened during this interaction in order to elininate generalities on the part of the mother. In effect she was saying: "spell it out." It was pointed out to the mother that the choices for her son were not as broad as she specified.

Members of these families suffer from a sense of being unable to reach one another on a feeling level. Each person strives for relatedness, but feels that the others block his efforts, preventing intimacy or affection. This type of psychological distancing was apparent in this family. Mrs. S. insisted that her husband "just didn't understand." She attributed this to his lack of education because he had to work at an early age. Steve never felt free to discuss anything with his father. He feared a rebuff and yet desired closeness.

The need to present family solidarity to the outside world is great and may be described as a kind of collective family face-saving imperative. During the second visit, the mother challenged the statement that her "son's illness" was a family problem. She intimated that it could be his fault. Besides, the illness was nothing more than a readjustment to civilian life.

She said: "We never did have fights — oh, little things would come up now and then. But, we'd sit down and talk about them." Mrs. S. also claimed that the family relationship was harmonious and said: "We've had a wonderful marriage."

This statement illustrates the category suggested by Jackson and Lederer's phrase: the "gruesome twosome."[6] Individuals grow old together in an unsatisfactory marriage that is quite stable because neither is able nor willing to acknowledge his dissatisfaction.

Anger and hostile feelings are practically excluded from this family structure. When the nurse injected the statement that anger is a reality and should be expressed, preferably in words rather than actions, the family members nodded their heads. In response to the question: "How does the family express anger?", this interaction followed:

Mr. S.: I don't have anything to get angry about. I don't bother anybody.

Mrs. S.: I get in the car and drive around for an hour, not recklessly.

[6]Lederer and Jackson, p. 153.

Steve: I clam up — walk away — go to the mountain and practice shooting.

Nurse: How does the other guy know you're angry?

(Silence.)

When such angry feelings intrude themselves in the child's awareness, and he has no means for direct communication, he is apt to have a psychotic break as he moves into later adolescence or adulthood.[7]

When family psychological boundaries have few openings into emotionally significant extrafamilial experiences, the child will have difficulty in recognizing and interpreting a variety of feelings and experiences. Growth is constricted in this type of family structure. The child is prohibited from engaging in interpersonal experiences. As a result of this, he will be lacking in adaptive mechanisms that are so essential for social adjustment. This situation was evident throughout Steve's schooling. He felt inferior to the students and refrained from establishing friendships. He argued with the teachers, refusing to follow through on their assignments, because he thought they were "stupid and ridiculous." As an enlisted man in the military service, he strongly desired to have his ideas accepted, instead of those from his superiors. He was totally unprepared to accept the bureaucracy that exists in the military.

The intensity and duration of pseudomutuality in this family has led to the development of shared mechanisms. Wynne calls them indiscriminate approval and secrecy.[8] These mechanisms tend to exclude from recognition or to reinterpret delusionally any deviations from the family role structure. They contribute to a failure by the potential schizophrenic in learning to discriminate who he is or where he is, except in terms of a blurred place in the family role structure. Failure to differentiate himself from the role structure signifies that the structure is encompassing.

Indiscriminate approval is given to a youngster even though this conflicts with the values of the family. Mrs S. often remarks: "We only want Steve to do what he wants to do." In this situation, it is difficult to be aware of disturbed behavior. To exemplify this mechanism when Steve was admitted to a military hospital for projective psychological testing, he wrote letters to his mother, telling her all was well and he was temporarily admitted to the hosital. She assumed that "all was well" and made no further inquiry.

Secrecy was another mechanism employed by the S. family. During one session a suggestion was made to the family members that they talk about a topic of controversy in the family. The three topics discussed

---

[7]Lyman C. Wynne, "Some Indications and Contraindications for Exploratory Family Therapy," *Intensive Family Therapy,* New York, Harper & Row, 1965, p. 303.

[8]Lyman C. Wynne, "Pseudo-Mutuality in the Family Relations of Schizophrenics," *The Family,* The Free Press, 1968, p. 634.

were gun control, the Vietnam war, and the campus riots. When asked if the family members had ever discussed personal problems, the mother retorted: "These are personal things that we don't share with anyone."

The ability to make decisions is nonexistent in the pseudomutual structure. This was especially significant during the time that Steve was a hospital patient for a "drinking problem." His mother visited him at the hospital. When questioned by the nurse, during a therapy session, whether she knew what was wrong with Steve, she replied negatively. She offered several excuses, such as the doctor didn't tell her anything, or they were still taking tests, or the doctor was nice, or they allowed her the free run of the place. She was incapable of deciding to ask about her son. This characteristic of pseudomutuality is quite common in general hospitals as well. A parent brings a youngster to the hospital for a surgical procedure. In many instances she has not prepared the youngster or the other siblings (in the event of a deformity). She waits, unable to make a decision. She will usually circulate around the room and enter into a conversation with another patient.

The family role structure and the shared mechanisms are internalized by the child. Identification with the parents and internalization of the parental codes are important for the child's ego and superego. Also internalized are the ways of thinking, meaning, anxiety, confusion, and distortion.

A child who grows up in a setting that harbors contradictions, develops certain perceptual capacities, especially when these contradictions are considered nonexistent. He will then consider his emotional responses unreliable towards understanding the expectations he has of himself and others. Furthermore, he will be incapable of understanding his own intrapsychic states: anger, resentment, disappointment. This would produce a panic situation as he becomes overwhelmed with anxiety, when approaching individuality. This can also be compared with the individual's moving out from the family role structure, resulting in an acute schizophrenic crisis. The psychotic break represents a futile attempt to achieve individuality.

Differences have been drawn here between solidarity and pseudomutuality. In the former, a feeling of mutuality exists. There is greater freedom for the individual to grow through experiential modes. Pseudomutuality is a stifling structure that constricts autonomy. It consists of ambiguity, meaninglessness, and emptiness. The family structure is compared to a familywide symbiotic ego. Individuality poses a great threat, especially with family members who have poor ego structure to begin with.

During therapy sessions, effort is directed at recognition of patterns and intervention. How does one intervene in this system to help towards reversing a pathological pattern that has been functioning for at least 30 years? First, there must be agreement on the part of the family that there is a felt discomfort, a disruption, or a desire for change. Second, strategies are directed at making former covert mechanisms a now-overt process. Attention is called to incongruities. Acting out of recent problems is requested. Members are urged to verbalize their anger. The family is reminded that a sick member is merely a signal that something is wrong with the system. Mention is made that whatever is wrong is going on in the family to perpetuate the difficulty.

More family therapy sessions will be required before a great deal of movement will be clearly discernible. However, an indication of growth, heard early in the sessions by a member of the family and repeated later was: "I do believe that family members hurt each other unwittingly."

BIBLIOGRAPHY

Bell, Norman W. and Ezra F. Vogel. "Toward a Framework For Functional Analysis of Family Behavior," *The Family,* New York, The Free Press, 1968, pp. 25–28.

Boszormenyi-Nagy, Ivan and James L. Framo. *Intensive Family Therapy,* New York, Harper & Row, 1965, pp. 13, 14, 64, 80, 302, 424, 450, 477.

Cousins, Albert N. "The Failure of Solidarity," The Family, The Free Press, N.Y., 1960, pp. 403–16.

Lederer, William J. and Don D. Jackson. *The Mirages of Marriage,* New York, W. W. Norton & Co., Inc., 1968, pp. 88, 153.

Wynne, Lyman C. "Pseudo-Mutuality in the Family Relations of Schizophrenics," *The Family,* New York, The Free Press, 1968, pp. 628–649.

12.

Amorphous Communication in a Family with Teenagers

Sister M. Rosalie Whalen

Early in a series of eight family therapy sessions with an assigned family, the writer noted that parental regulations for two teenage children were seldom clearly stated. However, following each instance of vaguely stated rules, parents conveyed expectations of high performance; there was low tolerance for failure to conform to parental standards. This recurring pattern of interaction within the family was identified as "amorphous communication."

In this selection, amorphous communication develops because of the following reasons:

1. Regulations are not clearly stated (by parents to teenage children).
   a. Regulations are vaguely stated regarding teenagers behavior.
   b. Confusion exists regarding successful role performance.
2. Teenagers try to attempt to fulfill role requirements.
3. Teenagers are unable to succeed.
4. Blame and disqualification of role performer's attempts are placed by parents.

Abstracts of data from family therapy sessions are included to illustrate the effect of amorphous communication on adolescent role performance in the family visited. The family consisted of Mr. M., father; Mrs. M., mother; Sue, daugher, age 15; and Lee, son, age 14.

The communication problem in the family appeared to be exacerbated by the fact that the two children were adolescents. A problem of great concern during the adolescent years revolves around the "drive for emancipation and independence."[1] Solution of the problem, according to Arieti, is largely dependent on affording the opportunities for self-

[1]Silvano Arieti, *American Handbook of Psychiatry,* Vol. I, New York, Basic Books, Inc. Publishers, 1959, p. 879.

direction and decision making, in gradually increasing amounts during the latency period.

The only specific reference to amorphous communication in the literature reviewed was made by Wynne, who defined the concept as "a vague, undirected form of communication."[2] Wynne regarded amorphous communication as a kind of family problem for which family therapy was possibly indicated. Family members, he pointed out, "are not so much afflicted by frankly contradictory, double-binding expectations but rather by vaguely defined expectations. Statements are not made and then disqualified but are instead never clearly enough stated so that one would know when a disqualification had occurred."[3]

Mrs. M.: Well I just feel you were very thoughtless. You were told not to be gone long and you said, "I won't be gone long," yet you were.

Sue: The reason I was gone so long was because Mary came along and then Rita. Rita is new here and we showed her around.

Therapist: What do you mean by long? Does Sue know what long means?

Mrs. M.: I'm sure she would say long to her is not the same as long to me.

Th.: But did you say how long?

Mrs. M.: No, I didn't say 2 hours, 30 minutes, or anything like that.

The above interaction was sufficiently typical to illustrate that in this family, rules or expectations weren't clearly stated. Hence whether or not a specific act is a violation is also not clear.

Laing, while describing a process similar to amorphous communication, used the term "mystification" and explained the concept in greater detail. According to Laing, mystification consisted essentially in "disguising, masking . . . or befogging the issues."[4]

As predicted theoretically, vague, indefinite expectations seemed to produce confusion in Sue and Lee as to what parents would consider satisfactory performance.

Mrs. M.: When you speak as you spoke right now, "I'm sorry" doesn't mean anything except a few words coming out of your mouth.

Sue: At times when I've said, "I'm sorry," you told me, That's all you ever say.

Th.: (to Mrs. M.) I'm not clear. What are you saying you want Sue to do to show she is sorry?

Mrs. M.: To say, "I'm sorry," at the time — not to wait until it's brought

[2]Lyman C. Wynne. "Some Indications for Exploratory Family Therapy," *Intensive Family Therapy,* New York, Harper & Row, 1965, p. 304.
[3]Ibid.
[4]Ronald D. Laing. "Mystification, Confusion, and Conflict," *Intensive Family Therapy,* New York, Harper & Row, 1965, p. 347.

up or she's more or less forced to say, "I'm sorry." Sue won't do this *even after she's cooled down.*

Th.: Sue just told Lee she was sorry about the incident Friday night.

Mrs. M.: Does it take her three days to cool down?

During the second family session, a contract was negotiated between Mrs. M.and Sue. Briefly, Sue was to clean her room on Saturday in return for which Mrs. M. agreed not to "nag" at Sue about her room.

Th.: How did the contract work out?

Mrs. M.: She supposedly cleaned her room Saturday without being told. I didn't check it because we were busy and had other things going.

When queried, Sue reported an attempt to fulfill her part of the contract. In this instance, it was impossible to confirm satisfactory performance because of failure to check the room. This was especially meaningful because the daughter's "disorderly" room was a prominent issue in two previous sessions.

In the following situation, Sue indicated she was unable to reproduce feelings experienced as a child. Hence, performance was unsatisfactory.

Mrs. M.: I don't expect her overnight to be what she was when she was younger.

Th.: What do you mean to "be like what she was when she was younger?"

Mrs. M.: To come up and want to be loved, to be hugged, and held tight.

Sue: Right now I don't know if I love anyone.

Amorphous communication or mystification may be used in such a way that one's own motives and intentions are discounted or minimized and replaced by others. "His experiences and actions . . . are construed without reference to his own point of view."[5] In short, there is blame and disqualification of the role performer's attempts. When teenagers make increased efforts at clarity, one or both parents respond negatively, thus serving to reinforce the old rather than the new ways.

Th.: How did things go since Thursday?

Mr. M.: Poorly.

Th.: Can you explain?

Mr. M.: The better communication between the children may have gone to a point where they're getting their heads together on positions to take in opposing us or at least Sue may be feeding some ideas to Lee.

[5]Laing, op. cit., p. 350.

SUMMARY

Amorphous communication and its impact on role performance as seen in one family setting has been described. It is an impossible task, particularly for teenagers, to fulfill expectations when regulations were not clearly stated.

Hammer has remarked that "Most of the adolescent's rebellious behavior is really a means of showing his parents that he is not a child and that he is capable of making independent decisions."[6] This observation has been validated by this family. Rigid parental control at a time when their children were demanding more independence seemed to precipitate a crisis situation in the family. This is a trying period for most parents but especially difficult for those who tend to be overprotective and unwilling to allow a testing of the adult role. A favorable resolution of the crisis for the M. family seems to depend on the parents' willingness to include their adolescent children in the decision-making function of the family.

BIBLIOGRAPHY

Arieti, Silvano. *American Handbook of Psychiatry,* Vol. I, New York, Basic Books, Inc. Publishers, 1959.

Hammer, S. L. and Jo Ann Eddy. *Nursing Care of the Adolescent,* New York, Springer Publishing Company, 1966.

Laing, Ronald D. "Mystification, Confusion and Conflict," *Intensive Family Therapy,* New York, Harper & Row, 1965.

Wynne, Lyman C. "Some Indications for Exploratory Family Therapy," *Intensive Family Therapy,* New York, Harper & Row Publishers, 1965.

[6]S. L. Hammer, and Jo Ann Eddy, *Nursing Care of the Adolescent,* New York, Springer Publishing Company, 1966, p. 54.

13.

Mistrust, Miscommunication, and the Malady Called Marriage

Aurelia Sue Kennedy

So they were married – to be the more together –
And found they were never again so much together,
Divided by the morning tea,
By the evening paper,
By children and tradesmen's bills.

Louis MacNeice:
Les Sylphides

I. THERAPY FOR THE TURMOIL OF TOGETHERNESS

New to the field of psychiatry is a perceptual framework through which individuals are seen in a relational perspective. No longer does the therapist probe for the "why" behind behavior, but the way in which all system members form interpersonal relationships and what strategies are used for their maintenance. Underlying this change has been the increasing focus on the dynamics of interpersonal relationships and the ensuing flux of material on systems. Paramount in this process is the switch from trying to "cure" the individual to exploring his continuing modes of behavior when confronting his fellow man. This phenomenon may be directly encountered in the field of family research and family therapy.[1]

Viewing a family as a system is clearest when one actually observes the dialogue of family members. In any home, it is obvious how each inhabitant influences the others in his system and how they influence him.

[1]Gerald H. Zuk and Ivan Boszormenyi-Nagy, eds., *Family Therapy and Disturbed Families*, California, Science and Behavior Books, Inc., 1969, p. 12.

Stability in the patterning of behavior evolves from the ongoing interactional processes. Primarily each one in the system reacts toward others in a mode that will beget pleasure and evade pain. The therapist cannot adequately explain the behavior patterns of any one member without careful scrutiny of how that member relates to those within his home and they to him.[2]

A beginning point for the study of a family as a system is to look at the types of relationships that are formed in a marriage. Lederer and Jackson refer to the type of relationship in which each spouse struggles for continuous equality as a symmetrical one. The message inherent in this kind of relationship is "I am as good as you are." Almost opposite in nature is the complementary relationship in which one spouse is in command and the other in submission to that command. In a marriage situation most relevant to our culture, one spouse is usually in command for certain aspects of the relationship, while the other spouse has other spheres of command. Most desirable and somewhat of a rarity is the parallel relationship in which the spouses respond to varying confrontations with alternating roles of symmetry and complementarity. When there are conflicting events, each spouse, perceiving of himself as equal to the other, will be both sustaining and at variance without fear, realizing that each will have his turn in victory of an issue. Basic to the formation of a parallel relationship is the establishment of trust, a resultant phenomen of honesty and openness in dealing with agreements and disagreements wherein each spouse is aware of his standing with his mate.[3]

Common to the institution of marriage is discord concerning what rules to observe in relating to one another, what kind of relationship to establish, who is to determine the rules, and when and the resolution of dealing with the incompatability between the rules. Furthering the discord may be an incongruence between the method for dealing with discord and the discord itself.[4]

Undeniably important in the task of the family therapist is identification of the various kinds of discord in a marriage and strategic interventions designed to alleviate the discord. From the very first hour of therapy, the family is invited to discuss their problems, become aware of the possibility for constructive change, and understand how their difficulties began and are perpetuated. Coupled with this invitation is the point that desirable growth is not the product of self-ventilation, clarifying disagreements, and discovery of the "whys" of their discord but a willingness on their part to take action to bring about a change.[5]

[2]Alfred Baldwin, *Theories of Child Development,* New York, Wiley, 1968, p. 540.
[3]William Lederer and Don Jackson, *The Mirages of Marriage,* New York. W. W. Norton & Company, Inc., 1968, p. 161.
[4]Jay Haley, *Strategies of Psychotherapy,* New York, Grune and Stratton, 1963, p. 128.

Supposedly basic to the marital state is that each partner must love the other. The understanding of what it means to love is one of the primary areas of difficulty in many families. True love is a difficult endeavor requiring more than most individuals are prepared or willing to give. Sullivan gives this definition of love: "When the satisfaction or the security of another person becomes as significant to one as to one's own satisfaction or security, then the state of love exists."[6]

It is not necessarily true that people marry for love. Often they enjoy the thought of themselves as loving and being loved, but all too frequently the emotion they believe to be love is in actuality another emotion such as sexual desire, insecurity, or an excessive need for acceptance. There are interesting and varied reasons for two people deciding to marry:

1. There is a loss in ability to reason astutely during courtship.

2. There is a cultural bind toward the state of marriage.

3. There is undue and hasty pressure from parents.

4. There are unrealistic values imposed on marriage by "romantic literature, tradition, and social hysteria" which the highly emotional couple design to be correct.

5. There are frequent marriages between lonely people.

6. There is a fear regarding their financial developments.

7. There is a desire to raise their status or socioeconomic level.

8. There is a purposeful selection of a neurotic partner to maintain a neurosis.

9. There is a need for a partner who will be a parent for them.[7]

To build a marriage that can be mutually satisfactory to both partners, there must be four building blocks: "tolerance, respect, honesty, and the desire to stay together for mutual advantage."[8] It would be a difficult endeavor to attempt to uphold a marriage founded on love unendingly. Equally as impossible is living in an unfoundering state of romance. It is normal and expected that love will not be continuously unwavering. Marriages that appear to last the longest may entail love only 10 percent of the time, and are based on respectful treatment of one another with unfolding opportunities and pleasures for each.[9]

Real communication in a family hinges from a significant depth of trust among the members. One can uphold an enduring openness to the other's needs only if one can trust that the other will possess the same openness.

[5]*Ibid.*, pp. 136, 137.
[6]Lederer and Jackson, *op. cit.*, p. 42.
[7]*Ibid.*, pp. 42-46.
[8]*Ibid.*, p. 56.
[9]*Ibid.*, p. 59.

A family system in its entirety can be molded by the permeation of dissolution of an environment of trust.[10]

Trust may be defined as:

confidence in or reliance on some quality or attribute of a person or thing, or the truth of a statement. Also: the quality of being trustworthy; fidelity; loyalty; trustiness. To trust means to have faith or confidence that something desired is or will be the case and to invest with a charge; to confide or entrust something to the care or disposal of the other.

Trust in marriage is established when the verbal and nonverbal behavior are consistent. It evolves from interchanges that are lucid among the family members. It occurs as an eventuality of a pliant, sequential bargain between spouses that lasts because they are able to adjust to the new and unexpected. The word trust originally stems from the Scandinavian language and meant "to comfort, to console, to confide in." Families who trust have learned to expect certain behavior from other family members because the past has taught them that their affiliation entails reoccuring phenomena. Today's usage of the word does not necessarily imply consoling and nurturing behavior because comforting another human being may be alien to the personality, past, beliefs, and goals of one who trusts. When family members are honest with one another and attempt to communicate clearly, the bonus may well be mutual generosity, confiding, and support. Trust is not formed from the kind of honesty where one spouts forth a belief, but on the kind where one does what is promised. Inherent in the development of trust is the requirement that it be a mutual possession of all family members; the family member who "trusts" an uncaring (thus undependable) member is usually a vain, frightened person — not one who trusts. Last, trust must abound on the continuous operation of mentation, veracity, and valor.[11] Operationally defined, trusting involves these sequential steps.:

1. There is a mutual need for respect within a system.

2. There is a system awareness of this need.

3. Trusting is a way to meet the need for mutual respect.

4. Each family member choses one or more members of the system in which to have faith. (Something is entrusted.)

5. The individual in the system has expectations that the faith will be honored.

6. He places himself in a position of vulnerability.

7. The faith is honored (i.e., the vulnerability is tested).

[10]Ivan Boszormenyi-Nagy and James L. Framo, eds., *Intensive Family Therapy,* New York, Harper & Row, 1965, pp. 83, 84.

[11]Lederer and Jackson, op. cit., pp. 106, 107, 109, 111-113.

8. Respect is thereby given and that aspect of the system functions productively.

9. Trust is established in the system.

or

7. The faith is betrayed (i.e., the vulnerability is retracted).

8. Respect is not given and that aspect of the system functions detrimentally.

9. Mistrust is established.

Were marital partners to achieve full benefit from their adventure, their vows to one another would be something as follows:

We have voluntarily agreed to form a marital partnership for our mutual benefit. We are human beings, and will grow and change with age and circumstances. Neither of us is perfect. We are not afraid of being fallible and therefore we will be honest and open with each other, and reveal ourselves and our changes or failures; we will disclose the hidden things when they unexpectedly emerge from the unconscious or from the forgotten past. If what happens is joyful (as we have faith it will be most of the time), we will treasure this good fortune. But if events are painful or harmful, we will adjust and accept the change because it is a fact. Instead of exhibiting frustration and being punitive toward each other, we will be consoling and encouraging. We will discuss realistically whatever has happened and see how it relates to us mutually, and as equals, we will decide what action is required. We also will discuss, if necessary, how both of us may change or adjust for our mutual benefit. More important than ourselves as individuals is our marital compages.[12]

II. MISTRUST, MISCOMMUNICATION, AND MEANINGFUL MANEUVERS

One of the most prevalent methods for perpetuation of mistrust in a family system is the accompanying miscommunication. Mistrust need not be formed on the basis of disapproved behavior alone but on the styles of relating that are characteristic of the system. Such a family where mistrust is the dominant theme of many an interaction is that of Frank and Maria Harper. Both have had previous marriages, and in the present family system there are two daughters from Maria's first marriage, and a son from the husband's first marriage. Before they met some five years ago, Frank was studying for a master's degree in theater and drama in Los Angeles and lacked one quarter for meeting graduation requirements. On

[12]*Ibid.,* p. 112.

a trip, Frank met Maria, and after six months they married and settled down. While he somehow made her believe that he was no longer interested in theater work and would accept a job with more-regular hours, it was not long after the marriage that he resumed his activity in the theater. Recently the marriage was shaken by a series of failures on Frank's part when he attempted to return to school in Los Angeles, attempted to operate a motel, and attempted social service work but failed because of a drinking problem and unorthodox approaches to his work. Presently he is involved with part-time theatrical work and a job as a service station attendant. Maria maintains a job as a waitress, which results in conflicting hours for opportunities to be together. Their marriage is characterized by what Jackson and Lederer call the unstable-unsatisfactory pattern.

In the unstable-unsatisfactory pattern the spouses are able to impart some information, but it is inadequate, frequently inexpedient, or cognitively chaotic, and unexpected information put into the system (frequently by the children) causes uproar. It seems impossible for the couple to share a viewpoint without engendering a fight or psychosomatic episodes, but they still expound their ideas even in the disturbance. All too often the children are the victims of scapegoating or being caught in the middle of a "war" on who is right. The children sometimes develop a diplomatic wisdom prematurely for their age, and this quality sometimes creates a gulf between them and their peers, which makes them feel "lonely, different, and vaguely inadequate."[13]

Those who endure the unstable-unsatisfactory marriage are entitled the Weary Wranglers by Lederer and Jackson. Compounded on long years of battling is great skill in hurting one another often and well. When the marriage is not ended by desertion, suicide, or divorce, the spouses find increasing pleasure in observing the other make a mistake or encounter a failure. Each mistake and each failure are tallied as defeats in their ongoing battle.[14]

The indefiniteness of their future is partly based on the lack or knowledge and willingness to end the battling and begin to work out bargains. When a viewpoint is being given or an activity pursued, each is more concerned with winning than delving constructively into the present issue. Concomitant with the need for victory in every battle is an inability to stay on one issue until it is resolved. It is not uncommon to hear the focus change with each new sentence.[15]

The underlying motivation behind unstable-unsatisfactory couples not leaving one another is because each spouse dreams of receiving "unpaid

[13]*Ibid.*, p. 140.
[14]*Ibid.*, p. 140.
[15]*Ibid.*, p. 142.

emotional bills from the past." There is a clouded but enduring hope for what the other partner could do if he only would. The message each harbors is: "Someday he'll realize how I've been wronged and he'll be more loving and appreciative and then we can be happy."[16]

Further deepening the difficulties of Frank and Maria are the real differences in their personalities and aspirations. Frank appears to be confident, rather self-dedicated, and persistent in his attempts to realize his goal of having his own theater. He is creative and intense and rather independent in his need for love and affection. Maria, on the other hand, would like a husband less creative and more stable to offer her the security she will probably never find. She is quite dependent and requires frequent demonstrations of affection. Both have participated in various forms of therapy such as individual, group, couples, and weekend marathon therapy. But rather than giving them a realistic mode for handling their differences, those therapeutic modes appear to have merely given them food for intellectual indigestion and regurgitation. Steps toward resolution of an issue were not in their behavioral repertoire. The following passage from *Mirages of Marriage* rather aptly depicts Frank's life style:

People of this sort may be unwilling or unable to change or compromise their behavior to patterns and tastes, with the result that genuine relationships with them are impossible. The most individualistic people in any society are generally those least amenable to personal change or to the compromise of cherished goals or ideals. Such individuals are often called loners and may be highly creative people or leaders, or they may be "outsiders," destructive rebels or hermits. (Frank appears to alternate between both *roles.) Unwillingness to compromise does not guarantee creative ability, but it is often characteristic of creative people. Many such people refuse to sacrifice the time, energy, or dilution of their central aims necessary to maintain a prolonged personal relationship.*[17]

Maria is characterized by portions of Satir's work. She frequently voices her fears, her anxieties, her insecure feelings, her need for attention, her dissatisfaction with life in general, and a feeling she often misterms "guilt." People with low self-esteem such as Maria obtain much of their feeling of worth from what others think of them. They are adept at hiding their low self-esteem from others, especially if there is an impression to be made. The foundation of the person with low self-esteem most probably stems from childhood experiences that left him feeling that it is undesirable to be an individual of one sex in relation to an individual of the other. Full separation from the parents has never been achieved as there remains an inequality in relationship with them. Underlying much of

[16]*Ibid.,* p. 147.
[17]*Ibid.,* p. 194.

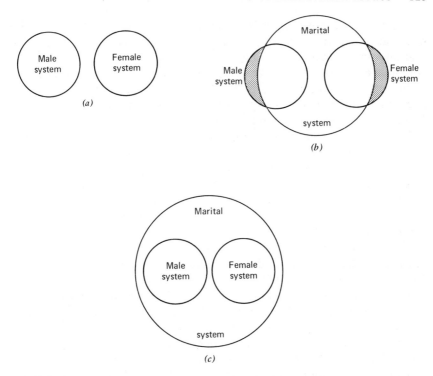

FIG. 1. Relationships between systems. (*a*). Before a relationship has developed. The two systems function independently. (*b*). After a relationship has developed. The more collaborative the couple, the smaller will be the portions (shaded) of their individual systems that function independently of the marital relationship system. (*c*). A near-perfect collaborative relationship.

the distress in Frank and Maria's marriage is the following facet wherein a person with low self-esteem has great expectations about what he can look forward to from others, but he is also plagued with fears; he is much too expectant of disappointment and so distrusting of those in his system.[18]

When this family began therapy, Maria had previously been labeled as the Identified Patient, another evolvement of an individual with low self-esteem. When that concept is threatened by some event of survival significance (such as Frank's series of failures), or some communication that implies, "You do not count; you are not lovable; you are nothing," the previously operative defenses break down and he develops more obvious symptoms that get him labeled "ill."[19]

[18]Virginia Satir, *Conjoint Family Therapy*, Palo Alto Science and Behavior Books, Inc., 1967, p. 8.
[19]*Ibid.*, p. 96.

Another illustrative example of how mistrust is maintained in this marriage is by the lack of respect for what Boszormenyi-Nagy calls "autonomous otherness." This is in evidence when family members complete each others sentences or attempt to reveal each other's deepest feelings. Lack of regard for the other's message is present. At first glance it might seem that the family is relating quite well (as did Frank and Maria's), but a closer examination will disclose the following:

The amorphous family organization may take the form of an ostensibly well functioning transactional system. Intersubjective sharing may deceptively appear as intensive relating. On closer observation, however, members of such families turn out to be incapable of genuinely reciprocal commitments to each other. They seem to selectively disregard messages and meanings that may be conducive to individuality and autonomous growth.[20]

The following diagrams better illustrate the concept of autonomous otherness and alludes to the difficulty couples encounter with the ideas of what is for "me" and what for "we." Figure 1 points out how marriage is:

A complex unity made up of at least three different but interdependent parts: the system of the male (his total being): the system of the female (her total being): and the marital system, deriving from the interaction of the male and female systems joined together (the compages, the relationship). The marital system springs into being spontaneously when the systems of male and female join. It is a good example of the whole being more than the sum of its parts, of one plus one equaling three.[21]

The operation of autonomy versus symbiosis in marriage necessitates steps for mutual understanding as the autonomous behavior of one partner may, if not clarified and agreed upon, leave the other feeling deserted and unwanted. In Figure 2, there are illustrations of various possible relationships between autonomous behavior (by one or both spouses) and the marital system itself.

(*a*) Part (shaded) of one spouse's system is operating autonomously independently of the marital system, and the non-autonomous spouse is left at home feeling abandoned.

(*b*) Part (unshaded) of each spouse's system is operating in symbiosis with the other; the remainder (shaded) is operating autonomously, independently of the marital system.

(*c*) An increment (blackened area) is added to each spouse's autonomy by a well-functioning marital system. Functioning well, however, depends on each being equally autonomous. A feeling of abandonment would occur if one began to be more autonomous than the other; this could

[20]Boszormenyi-Nagy, *op. cit.*, pp. 65, 66.
[21]Lederer and Jackson, *op. cit.*, p. 188.

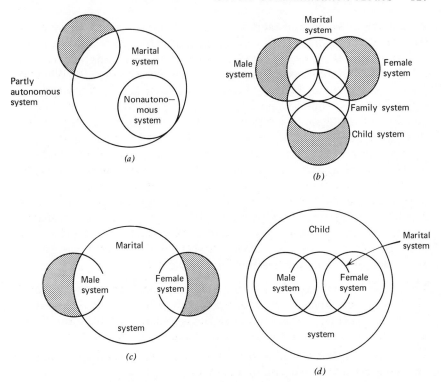

FIG. 2. Possible relationships between autonomous behavior and the marital system.

escalate into competition as to who could be more autonomous, and end in separation or divorce. When functioning well, this is a picture of an "egalitarian" family, in which both parents and child (ren) function autonomously to some degree, but parts of their systems operate in symbiosis. "Togetherness" provides room for independent growth for all.

(d) The extreme example in which the child's system engulfs both parents' systems and the marital system, so that the child's system dominates any autonomy the parents have in relation to each other. In this case, the parents compete for the child, and if one gains unequal favor with the child, the other feels abandoned or rejected by both spouse and child. If there are several children, each parent may "choose" one, so that the family may split into multiple coalitions.[22]

A family member with low self-esteem, such as Maria, experiences autonomous behavior as a differentness that signifies a conflict of plans. As a result she sees a move toward autonomy as an insult and evidence

[22]*Ibid.*, pp. 190-191.

for not being loved. Had each member of the dyad more self-esteem, he would be able to trust the other, feeling confident in reciprocal action, being able to wait, giving to the partner without feeling cheated, and viewing the differentness of the other as a prelude to growth. When two people lack trust they give conflicting messages that say: "I am nothing. I will live for you." and "I am nothing, so please live for me." In the couple who cannot trust, such as Frank and Maria, certain areas of joint living that beckon an attempt to realize the individual as a separate being are exceptionally foreboding to them. These areas are money, food, sex, recreation, work, and child rearing. To introduce trust into their system, it is necessary for them to decide what they will share and what they will not (those areas for dependence and independence). There has to be a balance between what each wants, does best, and thinks. From that can be negotiated the realm of responsibilities. The difficulty in clarification of areas for autonomy, decision making, and the disregard for the inherent messages is illustrated in the following clinical data:

Frank: I do want to go to Los Angeles later. Actually I had always worked up until two months ago. I guess I really don't know what I want to do. I've been directing a show for the Harkness Studio, but they don't really need me now, so I need to make a decision about what to do next.

Maria: What I really want to work on is your fear. I feel very insecure, and have great fear that you may cop out.

Frank: Well, as I see it, the real problem in this family is that everybody just looks out for himself. We were that way when we all got together.

Their primary learning task is that of assertion of thoughts, wishes and feelings, as well as knowledge, without demolishing, ingressing, or canceling the other and meanwhile emerging with a bargain suitable to both. Were they to work out a functional relationship, their messages would imply: "I think what I think, feel what I feel, know what I know. I am being *me* but I do not blame you for being you. I welcome what you have to offer. Let us both see what we can work out that would be most realistic."[23a] Failing to achieve a functional relationship, the messages imply: "Be like me; be one with me. You are bad if you disagree with me. Reality and your differentness are unimportant."[23b] Lack of realistic expectations probably hamper Frank and Maria's marriage further. When they do not achieve the total agreement they once experienced, they are hurt and begin a pattern of accusing one another for the failure.[24] Another pattern in the Harper family that dissolves trust is the "teeter-totter syndrome" that they embark on frequently. In essence it involves name calling and arguments about who should do what when.[25] One therapeutic

[23a,b]Satir, *op. cit.,* pp. 13.
[24]*Ibid.,* pp. 14, 15.
[25]*Ibid.,* p. 17.

strategy for establishing differentness is to have the family members negotiate for times and ways to allow for their differentness. When differentness is denied or argued about, one frequent result is pathology in the children.[26]

One of the characteristic patterns for maintenance of mistrust in the Harper family is also a rotational system for labeling and scapegoating. In every session, another family member was focused on and labeled in some derogatory way. While it is painful for any family member to be so labeled or scapegoated, it is especially disruptive to the emotional growth of a teenager. The following clinical data illustrates the father labeling and scapegoating 13-year-old Marcia:

Maria: Saturday, I brought some brandy and during the weekend I had three drinks out of it, but I later noticed it was half gone, and this is what started it all. As soon as I brought it in I started getting bad vibrations from Marcia. She asked me why I brought the brandy, and I said because I like it. Well, anyway, I only had one drink Saturday, one yesterday, and one last night. Frank said he noticed that the bottle was almost full. I know your dad didn't drink it because he would have told . . . certainly told me if he had.

Marcia: Well, we certainly didn't do it either.

Frank: You're acting awfully smart, Marcia, like you think this is all one big funny game. Marcia, could Rand have done it? She knows she is not to have boy friends in the house when we are not here.

Marcia: But I didn't do it.

Frank: I don't believe you. One of you is lying — one or both of you. What the hell were you doing letting people come in while we are gone? What were you doing?

Marcia: There were two other kids here besides Rand and we just sat in the living room.

Nancy (sister): Tell him what you went in the kitchen for.

Marcia: We went into the kitchen to get a drink of water, but Nancy came in too.

Nancy: So you see, dad, we didn't do it!

Frank: How is it that I never can talk to Marcia without you defending yourself. I never can talk to Marcia — because you always jump in. I never can talk to Marcia because I never get to it.

Nancy: But you were accusing both of us of knowing something about it and we don't!

Frank: I wasn't accusing you, but one of you know, and one of you don't know.

[26]*Ibid.*, p. 104.

Therapist: Would you clarify that?

Frank: I said One of you know, and one of you don't know, but I'm saying that one of you *does* know.

Therapist: Marica, would you react to what he is saying?

Marica: I don't know how to react — I never do. (Silence followed for the remainder of the session.)

Ginott has the following ideas for how parents should relate to their teenagers and how this type of relationship as described below would enhance an atmosphere of mutual trust in the family:

When parents become aware of imperfections in themselves they are often tempted to impose perfection on their children. Some parents make a career of it. They ferret out unpleasant facts about their teenagers conduct, and track down small defects in his character. For his own good, so they believe, he needs to be reminded of his deficiencies. Such honesty eventually kills communication between parent and teenager. No one benefits from flaws flung in his face. It is too threatening for a teenager to cope with the naked reality of his personal faults. Calling attention to them is like shining a harsh spotlight on him. His imperfections will become clearer to us, but not to him. His eyes will shut instantly. It is not helpful to dwell on character flaws. When forced to admit such faults publicly, a teenager may no longer want to correct them privately. In situations in which flaws are apparent, our immediate task is to help him cope with present crises. Our long term task is to provide him with relationships and experiences that correct character and build personality. Our main purpose is to tempt him to live up to his human potential. This purpose is better implemented quietly than proclaimed loudly.[27]

Further light is shed on dealing with a teenager as Ginott would seem to be pointing a finger at Maria's tendency to suffer with and for the family members, as evidenced in this data:

(Prior to the mother's following statement, the focus had been on how Marcia withdraws and will not communicate when accused for some piece of behavior.)

Maria: I get furious! I get very afraid! Always before I felt Marcia didn't really have any problems, because her grades were so good in school. She seemed to like the way we lived in Allentown because we had a nice house and a nice car. But she said so little that we began to read her mind and speak for her. One time I followed her into the bathroom and said,

[27]Haim C. Ginott, *Between Parent and Teenager,* Ontario, The Macmillan Company, 1969, p. 35.

"Marcia, what do you want from us?" And she didn't say a thing. I felt so sorry for her that I began to cry out and gave her affection and hugged her, and knew she must feel terrible.

To this kind of behavior Ginott says:

To be helpful, we need to learn empathy — an ability to respond genuinely to our child's needs and feelings without being *infected* by them. We need to help our teenager with his anger, fear, and confusion, without ourselves becoming angry, fearful, and confused.[28]

Typical of the communication in the family are individual thought disorders. Irregular and disconnected styles of interaction are illustrated by "vague drifting of a discussion through shifts in the object of attention, blurring of meaning by using uncertain referents and irrelevant meanings.[29] Every message has at least three aspects: the report aspect, the command aspect, and the context aspect. If family members are to interact productively, the listener must "hear" all three aspects of the message appropriately. If the messages clash or are unconnected, the listener cannot "hear" what he is really supposed to attend to. When a disconnected message is emitted, the receptor must inquire as to the intended meaning before he can respond correctly.[30]

One frequently observed phenomenon of this type is observed in the Harper family as they frequently use the "incomplete transaction." One of the family members will make a statement to which he gets a response, and his reply contains the message that he was not understood. The interaction was not complete because each did not ask of the other what is really meant and further noncompletions occur. Frequently a statement has so many different messages in it that the family member realizes that to respond to any one of the messages will put him in conflict with the other parts. This interaction is common to the "unstable, unsatisfactory" family, for many issues are expounded but never resolved. In this situation neither the husband nor the wife will capably handle the problem of rights about the kind of relationship they have. Any issue that requires cooperation becomes a problem of "who will decide what" ending in repeated disharmony.[31]

Another type of incomplete transaction that leads to mistrust from its lack of clarity is the type where the listener hears only fragments of a thought and he must fill in the rest.[32] The following data illustrates this:

[28]*Ibid.*, p. 41.
[29]Elliot G. Mishler and Nancy E. Wexlar, eds., *Family Processes and Schizophrenia,* New York, Science House, 1968, p. 24.
[30]Lederer and Jackson, *op. cit.*, p. 217.
[31]Don Jackson, ed., *Communication, Family, and Marriage,* California, Science and Behavior Books, Inc., 1968, pp. 233, 234.
[32]Satir, *op. cit.*, p. 71.

Maria: Back when they were having the riots in Los Angeles Nancy got all involved and actually helped to distribute some of the literature and went to some of their meetings. And you know . . . well, you know how that is.

Therapist: No, tell me.

Maria: As I see it, it is a kind of status thing, an in-thing to do.

The incomplete transaction is again seen when an issue is being raised in the family and instead of dealing with the issue at hand, Maria begins to express feelings of sorrow and guilt, not really relevant to the solution of the problem. To further complicate it she overapologizes until the message seems to be an apology for her birth as well. What seems to be wanted is that everyone reply, "Oh, it's all right. Don't be sorry, you're right and I'm wrong. You poor dear, how could I have wronged you so?"[33]

Mistrust is further engendered when one who has poor communication techniques seems unable to perceive and interpret his own messages to himself or the listener. As a result, the assumptions from which he decides to act are incongruous and unsuitable.[34] For example:

Maria: He's told me that he is not going to accept help, that when he is going to school he does not want to feel obligated to me. He says he will not take my money. I heard him say this and this is how I want it.

Therapist: And you are saying that this makes you feel guilty?

Maria: I'm saying, this is how I want it. I guess guilty isn't the right word.

Therapist: What word would you say is right?

Maria: Well, I just don't want you (to husband) to feel like I'm doing you a favor — I'm doing it for all of us. That's what I want to do. I'm not obligated.

Therapist: If I heard you correctly, I thought you said he didn't want that. I don't understand how it is a favor if he doesn't want it.

Another frequently used style of communication in the family is what Jackson refers to as the "double bind concept." It:

Refers to a pattern of pairs or sets of messages, at different levels, which are closely related but sharply incongruent, occurring together with other messages which by concealment, denial, or other means seriously hinder the recipient from clearly noticing the incongruence and handling it effectively, as by commenting on it. Instead he is influenced toward incompatible behavioral responses while invited not even to notice either influence or incompatibility. . . .[35]

[33]Nora Johnson, "The Art of Apology," *Cosmopolitan, LXVII,* August, 1969, pp. 36-38.
[34]Satir, *op. cit.,* p. 92.
[35]Don Jackson, ed., *Therapy, Communication, and Change,* California, Science and Behavior Books, Inc., 1968, pp. 225, 226.

Although several of the family members were observed to implement a double bind, it is seen most frequently between the husband and wife that she appears to approve of something he has told her and at the same time tells him of her fears about it. She asks for the security of a regular job, but each attempt at securing one is always met with both approval and disapproval of some sort.

The family system becomes dysfunctional when a member uses a statement to deliver several conflicting messages, by way of several levels of interaction and utilizing different signals:[36]

Maria: (crying). You had coffee with Charles and time to talk with him for several hours. But if I woke you from your nap and said I wanted to talk with you, you would be grouchy. I needed you and wanted to talk to you and I knew I couldn't.

Frank: You are always coming out of an agreement. We have a standing agreement about how bad we each feel when we first wake up and that we won't talk. So, what did you need me for?

Maria: I just wanted to relax with you and visit with you for a little while.

Frank: Now, I'm hearing three or four messages. One is that you are angry with me for visiting all day. Another is that you are angry with me for sleeping all day. Another is about how much you needed me. And the last is how you had such a bad day at work.

Maria: I really needed rest. I wouldn't have gotten so upset if it hadn't been for staying out so late with you.

Frank: That is not a good enough answer. You have to help yourself where that is concerned, because you can always stay home.

Maria: Normally I wouldn't be so grouchy; this just doesn't sound like me.

Frank: I really don't know what is going on. You are feeling so bad, and coming on so strong.

Maria: Well, I feel you are really coming on pretty strong yourself. You are so sure of yourself and I'm scared.

Therapist: So which is the real message you want him to hear?

Maria: That I just wanted a little time with him before you came.

Therapist: When do you normally tak with him?

Maria: (crying harder). Well it seems like I never do. We haven't had a schedule for a long time. The way I see it my time is whenever he is ready to give it to me. And I just have to wait until the time is right, if it ever is.

Trust is again waylaid when a family member communicates in a fashion whereby he generalizes, operates from assumptions, and clouds

---

[36]Satir, *op. cit.,* p. 92.

the meaning of the issue at hand, making it difficult to get back to the original issue.[37] This is illustrated in the following interchange:

Frank: When I left Los Angeles, I was working on a masters' degree in theater and drama. I dropped out and decided to visit some friends and relatives for a while and ended up in Allentown. I did intend to go back and complete my degree, but, at this point, feel very uncomfortable about even trying again. With the Social Service Welfare Retirement Plan, I would have enough money to go back to school. What I don't feel is that I can take the responsibility on myself to go without her support. (Pause) I have stayed in Allentown and life has been pretty good, but I didn't really want to stay. What I do not see is the real reason for her not wanting to go as I had not fallen on my face at that time. Since then I have had three failures, but at that time I hadn't.

Maria: Well, my fears were centered around the way you were putting society, the Administration and everyone down. I thought you were terribly confused and didn't know what you wanted.

Frank: I thought she was projecting with nothing to go on. She didn't really have enough evidence at that time not to go.

Maria: I guess I just didn't want the responsibility of the world on my shoulders.

Further communication difficulties occur when one family member does not check out his perceptions of a situation to see if they are in agreement with the event as it actually is or with what the other person really meant.[38]

Maria: I was lying out in the sun Saturday and Nancy asked me to come in and show her how to make some vermicelli. I said no, that I wanted to lay in the sun. I came in in a little while to fix some lunch and told Bobby to wash his hands. He came back and it didn't look like he had washed them at all, so I took him in the bathroom and made him wash his face and hands. Then Nancy jumps on me and says he did wash his hands and I said, "Do you believe him or do you believe me?" Nancy said "Well, you didn't have to pull his hair." (Demonstrates how mother pulled hair turning his head and washing his face.) But I said I wasn't really pulling it, or, I don't think I was. Anyway, I feel Bobby will be very confused when he always hears her try to jump in and tell me what to do.

Making the interpretation of a situation from a past context is another example of poor communication and a means to the formation of mistrust:

Maria: Well, as I see it there are two things happening here. One is that Frank always checks with me before he will drink anything. Another is

[37]*Ibid.*, p. 71.
[38]*Ibid.*, p. 94.

that Marcia is not supposed to have any boyfriends here when we are gone. I realize I shouldn't have been, but I was really upset and full of fear that he had been drinking, so of course I asked him if he had.

The "here and now" is seen through labels fixed in the mind from the past, which negates the possibility of forming a new outlook on that issue.[39]

Another pattern is that of the "pseudobenevolent dictator" who imagines that he knows the needs and wants of the spouse without asking what the real needs might be.[40]

Maria: I really thought he was sick this past weekend. He should have told me he wanted attention. When I asked him if he needed some attention and love, he said, "No," he was "just exhausted from the tranquilizers."

Similar to that is mind reading, a pattern that cannot allow for development of trust since there is no real two-way mutual interchange:[41]

Maria: I really feel that Frank needs to talk more than we do. I feel that way because we met with you yesterday.

Frank: Oh, that's interesting that you think I need to talk, because it seems to me that everything that happened yesterday, happened after you grouped yesterday.

If two people are to successfully handle their problems, it must obviously be a joint enterprise. This joint effort becomes dissolved when the spouses begin to play the "if only" game, asking that one change before the other, and then the other will change. Frank and Maria are frequently playing this game, although Frank is more perceptive about how she is usually first to state the conditions of the "if only."[42]

Mistrust frequently occurs when Frank uses a "reverse vulnerability" technique for keeping distance between them. This term implies that he will not allow her to become too dependent of loving for fear that she will expect loving and nurturing behavior too often. He finds it difficult to decide when to be loving and when to try to retain his independence by withdrawal. This was illustrated in one session where he described her blocking him in the doorway for a kiss and he pushed her out of the way, saying that she was forcing him to love and he didn't want to. This pattern can only be broken by an assignment to take turns on deciding who will lead what with the other in full agreement. The lesson involved is that the giver becomes aware that giving need not be so degrading after all.[43]

---

[39]*Ibid.*, p. 93.
[40]Lederer and Jackson, *op. cit.*, p. 230.
[41]*Ibid.*, p. 226.
[42]*Ibid.*, p. 233.
[43]*Ibid.*, pp. 307, 308, 311-313.

III. STRATEGIES FOR INTERVENTION

The two primary interventions made with this family were to teach them how to negotiate successful *quid pro quos* and the use of the paradoxic intention. The *quid pro quo* is a necessary process for coming to a mutually satisfying agreement about an issue that needs resolving. It is in essence a bargain wherein each tells the other what he would like or want, but not how the other should behave. To reestablish trust, this technique is necessary for:

Close, enduring human relationships depend on an interplay of behavior which signals to each spouse that whatever he receives has been forthcoming in response to something given. In other words, a quid pro quo *(something for something) agreement is in effect. To live in reasonable harmony the spouses negotiate with respect to their behavior and responsibilities. Perhaps this kind of relationship appears selfish and unromantic, yet in our view it is the single most required and most overlooked aspect of any marriage.*[44]

In essence a *quid pro quo* is little different from Maslow's concept of self-actualization where there is "transcendence of selfish and personal motivations, the giving up of lower desires for higher ones, increased friendliness and kindness, and decrease in hostility, cruelty and destructiveness (although decisiveness, justified anger and indignation, self-affirmation, etc. may well increase)."[45] Basic to the establishment of the *quid pro quo* are other tactics given to the family for successful fighting including such ideas as not cross-complaining, sticking to one issue, having equal and assigned times to complain, not mind reading, and not dragging in the past.

Underlying the approach to this couple, too, was Haley's paradoxical intention that implies that the therapist does not give advice to change and not disagree and fight as they do but says, instead, for them to continue it. What happens with this approach is that when the couple do what they usually do under the direction of the therapist's orders they become more aware of their actions, and the disagreeing behavior is gradually modified to the establishment of workable *quid pro quos*. As a result, they are both forced and freed at the same time. Coupled with this permission to continue fighting, they are taught techniques for identification sequences of behavior, unveiling the real messages and relabeling of what they actually do.[46]

---

[44]*Ibid.*, p. 286, 304, and 17.

[45]Abraham Maslow, *Toward a Psychology of Being,* Princeton, New Jersey, D. Van Nostrand Company, Inc., 1968, p. 158.

[46]Haley, *op. cit.*, pp. 147, 148, 189.

IV. SUMMARY AND CONCLUSIONS

Therapy in this family was an attempt to help them be aware of their communicational techniques and how to change them to achieve happier outcomes. The approach was based on the beliefs that everyone is really geared to growth, that no one person is to be identified as the one at fault but as a symptom of distress in the system, and that one must free oneself of cognitive feelings to learn to actually validate with others what they perceive and come to real understandings.[47] As Satir sees it, man is in a continual conflict of wanting always to be loved and at the same time in power, and the only way to resolve the conflict is to allow them to coexist in the proper time and place so that each enhances the other. He can either war with his mate about who and what is right or can handle their differentness on the basis of "exploration and what fits."[48]

Basic to it all was a willingness to change on the part of every family member, for without this commitment, little can be done by the therapist. With the commitment, it is then up to the therapist to make the proper use of that willingness. As Zuk puts it:

Some people prefer to sit alone with the inner voices of their past relationships, repeating sequences of (compulsive) acts according to some internal patterning; never assert themselves in differing from the other's point of view; or exploit every human encounter as an opportunity for hostile rather than trusting exchanges. Some of these people lead lonely lives. Others find partners who collude with them in building bad relationships. In any case, people have deep motivations for maintaining their internal or external relationships and commitments, because these mean very much to them. One's self obtains meaning through relationships that mean much to it. Emotional growth, on the other hand, hinges on one's capacity for relinquishing nonworkable relational commitments and substituting workable new relationships.[49]

When two people are under the influence of the most violent, most insane, most delusive, and most transient of passions, they are required to swear that they will remain in that excited, abnormal, and exhausitng condition continuously until death do them part.

George Bernard Shaw:
preface to Getting Married.

[47]Satir, *op. cit.,* pp. 96, 97.
[48]*Ibid.,* p. 90.
[49]Zuk, *op. cit.,* p. 70.

BIBLIOGRAPHY

Baldwin, Afred. *Theories of Child Development,* New York, Wiley, 1968.

Boszormenyi-Nagy, Ivan and James L. Framo, eds., *Intensive Family Therapy,* New York, Harper & Row, 1965.

Ginott, Haim C. *Between Parent and Teenager,* Ontario, The Macmillan Company, 1969.

Haley, Jay. *Strategies of Psychotherapy,* New York, Grune and Stratton, 1963.

Jackson, Don, ed., *Communication, Family, and Marriage,* California, Science and Behavior Books, Inc., 1968.

Jackson, Don, ed., *Therapy, Communication, and Change,* California, Science and Behavior Books, Inc., 1968.

Johnson, Nora. "The Art of Apology," *Cosmopolitan, LXVII,* August, 1969, pp. 36-38.

Lederer, William and Don Jackson. *The Mirages of Marriage,* New York, W. W. Norton and Company, Inc., 1968.

Maslow, Abraham H. *Toward A Psychology of Being,* Princeton, New Jersey, D. Van Nostrand Company, Inc., 1968.

Mishler, Elliot G. and Nancy E. Wexler, eds., *Family Processes and Schizophrenia,* New York, Science House, 1968.

Satir, Virginia. Conjoint Family Therapy, Palo Alto, Science and Behavior Books, Inc., 1967.

Zuk, Gerald H. and Ivan Boszormenyi-Nagy, eds., *Family Therapy and Disturbed Families,* California, Science and Behavior Books, Inc., 1969.

Part IV
SCAPEGOATING AND LABELLING PROCESSES

14.

The Label That Disables

Jo Ann McKay

The major premise of this selection is that the process of labeling in a family system will produce the behavior named.

Labeling is a part of the general concept of socialization. Norms are learned in the process of socialization. The individual gets his prescriptions, what he ought to do and be, and his proscriptions, what he ought not to do or be, during the socialization process.

A question raised here is this: Are the prescriptions and proscriptions that parents believe they are teaching their children the same as the ones that the children actually learn?

I. THEORETICAL BACKGROUND

The process of socialization has been operationally defined[1] as follows:

1. Appraisals are made by significant others of the "self."
2. Appraisals are repeated many times and form a pattern.
3. Incorporation of appraisals occurs.
4. Based on appraisals, behavior emerges to match.
5. With each era of development the self is open for reappraisal.

This famework is supported by a review of the literature.

Lemert[2] introduces the useful concepts of primary and secondary deviation. Deviant behavior is primary when it is occasional, symptomatic, or situational and is dealt with as a function of a socially acceptable role. It is when the deviant behavior stabilizes into a social role and becomes a way of life that the deviation is secondary.

[1]Shirley Smoyak, lecture, Advanced Psychiatric Nursing Workshop, The University of New Mexico, 1970.

[2]Edwin, M. Lemert, *Social Pathology,* New York, McGraw-Hill, Inc., 1951, p. 75.

It is seldom that one deviant act will provoke a sufficiently strong, societal reaction to bring about secondary deviation. Most frequently there is a progressive reciprocal relationship between the deviation of the individual and the societal reaction, with a compounding of the societal reaction out of the minute accretions in the deviant behavior, until a point is reached where ingrouping and outgrouping between society and the deviant is manifest. At this point a stigmatizing of the deviant occurs in the form of name-calling, labeling, or stereotyping.[3]

Most of the occasional rule breaking that goes on in a family is of the primary type and never develops beyond this stage. Why then, does some primary deviation progress to secondary deviation? According to Lemert it is because, and only when, the deviant behavior gets reinforced by the reactions of others.

Scheff[4] discusses the same phenomenon using different terminology. He says that the usual reaction to rule breaking is denial and that in these cases most rule breaking is transitory. In a small proportion of cases the reaction goes *the other way*, exaggerating and, at times, distorting the extent and degree of the violation. This exaggeration is called labeling.

The effect of labeling as a source of uniformity and stability of deviant behavior is clarified in the following quotation:

When societal agents and persons around the deviant react to him uniformly in terms of traditional stereotypes of insanity, his amorphous and unstructured rule-breaking tends to crystallize in conformity to these expectations, thus becoming similar to the behavior of other deviants classified as mentally ill, and stable over time. The process of becoming uniform and stable is completed when the traditional imagery becomes a part of the deviant's orientation for guiding his own behavior.[5]

Scheff also points out that deviance refers to particular acts labeled as norm violations and, furthermore, that deviance is "not a quality of the act the person commits but rather a consequence of the application by others of rules and sanctions."[6]

Although Scheff is talking about the process in relation to the mentally ill, it appears to be equally applicable to the family system. In other words, it is not so much what a family member does as what others say about the act that determines whether the behavior gets labeled "good" or "bad," normal or deviant. The deviance is stabilized by the labeling process.

Goffman[7] emphasizes the effect of role expectations. Assumptions are made regarding what an individual ought to be and when he displays

[3]Ibid., p. 76.
[4]Thomas J. Scheff, *Being Mentally Ill*, Chicago, Aldine Publishing Co., 1966, p. 81.
[5]Ibid., p. 82.
[6]Ibid., p. 33.
[7]Erving Goffman, *Stigma*, Englewood Cliffs, New Jersey, Prentice-Hall, Inc., 1963, pp. 3–5.

evidence of possessing an attribute that makes him different and less desirable, he is reduced in the perceiver's view. Such an attribute is a stigma. It constitutes a special kind of discrepancy between what is expected of a person and what he actually is or does. Goffman suggests "that not all undesirable attributes are at issue, but only those which are incongruous with our stereotypes of what a given type individual should be." Thus, a stigma is defined as "an undesired differentness from what we had anticipated."[8]

The attitudes that "normals" take toward a person with a stigma, and the actions taken in regard to him, involve various forms of discrimination that effectively reduce his life chances. "We tend to impute a wide range of imperfections on the basis of the original one."[8]

In the family as well as in larger society, members tend to react negatively to another member who does not behave according to what was expected of him, and a "bad" label is ascribed. But even more damaging is the generalizing effect of this "bad" behavior so that the labeled member is accused of "always" being "bad" and of doing related "bad" things without evidence of this being so.

A related concept is that of sanctions Gibbs[10] defines a sanction as a reaction to deviant behavior and proposes that in order for a negative (or positive) sanction to be effective it should be characterized by the following:

1. The reactor should perceive the reaction as an infliction of punishment (or a reward).

2. The intent of the reaction is to prevent norm violations (or to encourage conformity).

3. The object of the reaction should perceive the reaction as a punishment (or reward).

4. The reaction and reactor are socially approved.

These additional contingencies of intent and perception in particular are relevant to the original question posed.

As a interim step before the presentation of clinical data, a consideration of other possible reasons for labeling in a family may lend perspective. A few possibilities are:

1. Lack of knowledge. Family members may not realize the effects of what they do.

2. Stereotyping. This classifies events and makes life more livable. Otherwise, each event would have to be considered as a separate event; learning would not be possible.

[8]Ibid., p. 5.
[9]Ibid.
[10]Jack P. Gibbs, "Sanctions," *Social Problems*, p. 153.

3. Prejudices. This accomplishes the management of low self-esteem by the labeler.

4. Scapegoating. This detracts attention from other family conflicts.

5. Retribution. This expresses indignation.

It appears that when most parents use negative labels within the family, the intent is to eradicate the named behavior. They think this will happen and when it does not, they become confused and angry.

The following operational definition of the process of labeling was developed and will be used to guide clinical intervention:

1. Family norms, rules, and role expectations are operating.

2. Socializers within the family (persons on a higher power level, usually parents or oldest sibling) appraise the socializee's behavior, using (1) as a guide, in the following ways:
   a. By a positive appraisal of desired behavior.
   b. By a negative appraisal of undesired behavior.
   c. By meeting a negative appraisal of undesired behavior, resulting from family-system needs, with exaggeration, generalization, and/or expectation that the undesired behavior will continue.

3. The socializee, since in "down one" position (on a lower power level), believes he has no option but to accept the appraisal.

4. The socializee is more likely to accept the label when the appraisal is:
   a. More frequent.
   b. More intense.
   c. Made early (as behavior first occurs).

II. CLINICAL EXAMPLES OF PATHOLOGICAL LABELING AND INTERVENTION INTO THIS PATTERN

The White family included Mr. and Mrs. White, Lisa, age 12, Karen, 11, Kevin, 8, and Jamie, 7. The pattern of labeling was evident during the first family session and focused on the identified patient, Jamie. Jamie was labeled as follows: disobedient, disruptive in school, short attention span, likes the hurt animals, too close to males, doesn't like females, pinches girls, has nightmares, little fellow, little type, and Mutt (of Mutt and Jeff).

Within the second family session it became clear that the same labeling process occurred in relation to all the children. Kevin was named a worrier, a Jeff (of Mutt and Jeff), lazy, lackadaisical, tattletale, a dreamer, and different. Karen was labeled a loner, scatterbrained, a ding-a-ling, and a second mother to Jamie. Lisa was called a liar, disobedient, sarcastic, sassy, boy crazy, growing up too fast, a tease, wears make up like a

French whore, neglects her duties, and a baby-sitter. Any two children who were arguing about who was getting preferential treatment from the parents were called the Smothers Brothers.

By the third and fourth sessions the pattern carried over to the parents as well. The mother was labeled by herself as well as her husband as a wicked stepmother, a goody, a black sheep, sexy, Little Amber (of *Forever Amber*), top sergeant, a Leo-lionhearted, a backslider, uptight, and impulsive. The father was named mighty mouth (at work), doesn't talk much at home, shy, easygoing, a Libra peacemaker, a procrastinator, and a backslider.

The pervasiveness of the pattern is evident. From this plethora of name calling it was observed that one particular label was repeated more frequently than others so that a central theme emerged for each person. Jamie hurt animals, Kevin was different, Karen was scatterbrained, Lisa was growing up too fast, mother was impulsive, and father did not talk much at home. These most repeated labels suggested major family problems.

An example of the exaggeration of a negative appraisal is evidenced by Jamie's hurting animals being relabeled by the parents as a cruel streak, malicious behavior, and likely to lead to arson, robbery, murder, or worse.

Therapeutic intervention was planned for the family based on the theoretical understanding that labeling produces the behavior named. To say it another way, you get the name and then you get the game. The plan was to use a reinforcement approach, to replace a "bad" label with a "good" label.

A cognitive approach was chosen because both Mr. and Mrs. White demonstrated a high level of intelligence and motivation. The plan was discussed in a therapy session with just Mr. and Mrs. White.

PLAN OF CLINICAL INTERVENTION FOR PATHOLOGICAL LABELING

1. Teaching the parents the socialization process.

a. Find out what they already know about how children develop based on their own personal experiences, reading, and what they have learned from other people.

b. Using information they have introduced, present to them the process of socialization as operationally defined on page 00.

2. Emphasize that parents are in control of the situation.

a. Tell them that therapists recognize that they have the idea that they can do something to bring about a change in Jamie when they really put forth the effort.

  b. Give examples of this.

  "When Jamie was having difficulty talking, you took him to the speech clinic and his speech improved."

  "For a long time the neighbors wouldn't let their children play with him. Now they do. You did something."

3. Show them the way.

  a. Tell them to decide on one thing they want Jamie to do. Make sure that it is stated as a clear, positive attribute or behavior.

  b. Have them come up with four or five synonyms.

  c. Tell them to make a schedule for recognizing this new named behavior.

    1. How many times a day?

    2. When?

  d. Have them set up a check system to see that they do it as scheduled. They may write the schedule on a note card, keep it in a pocket, and check it off each time they comment on the attribute or behavior.

  e. Watch the outcome.

  f. Remind them to make no negative statements about the behavior.

  g. Tell them that it is simple and that it will work.

  This approach will work because the appraisers get a new view of the one appraised and come to accept it and the one appraised gets the behavior to match.

  A variation of this clinical intervention can be used with low socioeconomic families. By omitting step 1 and beginning with step 2.

  The next example highlights the effect of expectation of the labeled behavior.

  During a family session the cat jumped on the sofa, Jamie petted the cat, and put the cat on his lap. He held the cat for several minutes then:

Karen: Jamie, let the cat go!

Jamie: (lets go of the cat, spreads his arms out, wide, the cat stays quite still, on its back at that, and does not move) See, he won't go.

Karen: (five minutes later) Jamie, put the cat down, you're hurting him (in insistent voice).

Jamie: (again opens his arms, the cat still does not move) No, I'm not. See, he won't go.

Karen: You're not supposed to hold the cat.

Karen: (two minutes later) Jamie, you're squeezing the cat. He wants down!! (voice much louder)

  At this point the cat does begin to meow and Jamie lets the cat go.

Jamie: I didn't do nothing.

It appears that after three suggestions that he would hurt the cat, Jamie did squeeze the cat tighter and confirmed the expectation that he is a person who hurts cats.

Karen: (to therapist) He's not supposed to hold the cat, he hurts him.

Therapist: I noticed that Jamie held the cat for about ten minutes without hurting him.

Karen: He killed Kevin's fish.

Notice that the children have learned to label each other and Karen quickly switches to another example of Jamie hurting animals when in the present situation Jamie is defined as a person who does not hurt cats.

A better intervention would be: "Karen, you're a good observer. You are really tuned in to what everybody is doing. Back up and get the beginning of this event. What did you first notice about Jamie and the cat?" The purpose is to help Karen reconstruct what actually happened rather than telling her and clashing directly with her ideas. Also the therapist acts as a role model of one who recognizes positive behavior.

This final example is what Goffman describes as a discrepancy between what we expected of a person and what he actually is or does.

Lisa had been caught by her parents as she was trying to drive the family car at 1:30 A.M.

Therapist: What was your reaction at the time?

Mother: I couldn't believe it. It's not like my mental picture of her or what she should be.

There are three aspects of a role:

1. The way it is.
2. The way it should be.
3. The ideal way.

Intervention could best be directed to helping the mother spell out her expectations of what Lisa ought to be, to get each to recognize on which of the above aspects of role she is operating, and to help them decide which one will be most acceptable.

SUMMARY

It is recognized that there are many and varied causes of deviant behavior. The process of labeling has been presented as functioning in both the production and the extinction of deviant behavior in a family system. The problem seems common enough to warrant special consideration.

The treatment of deviance would be more effective it it made use of techniques which accord with the reasons for behavior: Where ignorance is the cause, education; where lack of ability is the difficulty, improved training; where motivation is the problem, a planned and deliberately executed program of manipulation of rewards and punishments to re-orient the individual to appropriate goals and behavior.[11]

The clinical intervention suggested in this paper for the family problem of labeling demonstrates one such program.

That families unwittingly reinforce negative behavior by labeling and produce the very behavior that they wish eradicated is a tragedy that could be prevented and can be changed. It can be changed because with each era of development, the self is open for reappraisal.

BIBLIOGRAPHY

Brim, Orville G. Jr. and Stanton Wheeler. *Socialization After Childhood: Two Essays,* New York, Wiley, 1966.

Garfinkel, Harold. "Conditions of Successful Degradation Ceremonies," *American Journal of Sociology, 61,* March 1956.

Goffman, Erving. *Stigma,* Englewood Cliffs, New Jersey, Prentice-Hall, Inc., 1963.

Gibbs, Jack P. "Sanctions," *Social Problems.*

Lemert, Edwin M. *Social Pathology,* New York, McGraw-Hill, Inc., 1951.

Scheff, Thomas J. *Being Mentally Ill,* Chicago, Aldine Publishing Co., 1966.

Smoyak, Shirley, William Field, and Grayce Sills. Lectures, Advanced Psychiatric Nursing Workshop, The University of New Mexico, 1970.

Webster's New Collegiate Dictionary, Springfield, Mass., G. and C. Merriam Co., 1956.

---

[11]Orville G. Brim, Jr. and Stanton Wheeler, *Socialization After Childhood: Two Essays,* New York, Wiley, 1966, p. 43.

15.

Scapegoating: A Process Continuing When Parents Divorce

Harriett E. Goodspeed

The phenomenon of scapegoating is as old as human society. Sir James Frazer, in *The Golden Bough,*[1] records numerous instances reaching back to antiquity of public scapegoating, human and others. He views the process of scapegoating as one in which "the evil influences are embodied in a visible form, or are at least supposed to be loaded upon a material medium, which acts as a vehicle to draw them off from the people, village or town."[2] The scapegoat's function is "simply to effect a total clearance of all the ills that have been infesting a people."[3] This phenomenon of scapegoating can also be dealt with at the level of a society, tribe, or a family system. This selection deals with scapegoating as the overt signaling within a family system. This pattern is fairly common and can be identified when, within a family unit, a group can achieve unity through the scapegoating of a particular member. "Thus the deviant within the group may perform a valuable function for the group by channeling group tensions and providing a basis for solidarity."[4]

The idea that the family is largely responsible for the emotional development and health of the child is widely acceptable in contemporary behavioral sciences. The greatest emphasis has been placed upon child rearing practices and the personality and past history of the mother as they relate to the mother-child relationship. Some attempts have been made to investigate the father-child relationship in terms of the personality and past history of the father. Even more recently, the acceptable concept is to scrutinize the interrelations of all individuals and family

[1]Sir James Frazer, *The Golden Bough,* New York, Macmillan Co., 1927, p. 562.
[2]Ibid.
[3]Ibid.
[4]Norman W. Bell and Ezra F. Vogel, *A Modern Introduction to the Family,* New York, The Free Press, 1968, p. 412.

behavior in terms of a family system. Ackerman[5] states this idea as having three dimensions:

1. The group dynamics of the family.
2. The dynamic processes of emotional integration of the individual into the family.
3. The internal organization of individual personality and its historical development.

The emotional system that characterizes a particular family system begins with the marriage of two personalities.

Therapist: What was the bond that led you to marry your ex-wife?

Mr. W.: I felt sorry for her. She had had an abortion and had attempted suicide.

Therapist: When the problem was resolved and you were married, what then?

Mr. W.: It was the same. I felt sorry about what had happened and wanted to be with her.

The contract between these two people was one of mutual dependency based on reciprocal or complementary needs. The relationship of these needs does not imply perfection. There can be much marital conflicting stemming from power struggles, dependency, deep-seated grudges, and rejections.

Therapist: How was the decision made for you to leave the service?

Mr. W.: I had always wanted to be a pilot. I passed all the tests, but when I was ready to leave for Kelly Field she insisted I resign or she would leave me and return to Germany.

"One cannot assume that because a marriage persists these problems are resolved. The struggles and tensions may persist throughout a lifetime often ramifying into parents' relationship with the children."[6] The marriage of Mr. and Mrs. W. lasted 18 years, and the foci of problematic areas were the solidarity of this family and the sexuality between them. But they skillfully manipulated the delegation of family roles and labeled the problem to be one of internal instrumentality.

There are many factors that render a child the most appropriate object to deal with family tensions. A child is in a relatively powerless position compared to adults. Because the child is in the developmental phase

---

[5]Nathan Ackerman, *The Psychodynamics of Family Life*, New York, Basic Books, Inc., 1958, p. 24.

[6]Nathan B. Epstein and William A. Westley, *The Silent Majority*, San Francisco, Jossey-Bass, Inc., 1969, p. 59.

where his personality is very flexible, he can be molded to adopt the role that the parents assign to him. "The selection of a particular child as the scapegoat is not a random matter, one child is the best symbol."[7] The conflicts that existed in Mr. and Mrs. W.'s marriage from the beginning were never resolved. Therefore, severe difficulties in the marital relationship created tension that was quickly displaced on to the first available and appropriate object — the first child. Since the first child was available for scapegoating, she was assigned to this role, and once assigned accepted and continued it. A child with a serious illness of disfigurement can also become the focus of the family problems.

Therapist: Do you recall anything unusual about Linda's childhood?

Mr. W.: Yes, when she was about four months old she had some serious physical illness. High fevers, dehydration, sometimes pneumonia developed. She was a sickly child for the first three or four years.

Another pattern for scapegoating can be linked to family resemblance or continuity of family characteristics. The Identified Patient in this family is the oldest female child.

Therapist: Who do the children resemble in appearance and personality?

Mr. W.: Linda looks just like her mother. There's something else I've always wondered about. The oldest girl in my wife's family always had some kind of mental illness — the grandmother, the mother (my ex-wife) and now Linda.

Ackerman[8] raises a question: Is there some specific correlation between types of prejudicial scapegoating in certain families and do specific intolerances of symbolically perceived qualities in the offspring lead to scapegoating?

Linda was also the scapegoat for her parents' childhood deprivations. In their respective families of origin they had shared certain anxieties in common. Collected clinical data reveals that Mr. W. came from a broken home and had little, if any, recollection of his own parents. He speaks harshly and berates his ex-wife's parents. The father was incestuous, and the mother did not want children. The family structure was rigid and cold. Postwar conditions in Germany made physical and educational requirements meager and limited.

The assumption that the scapegoating situation can be a triadic structure is demonstrated by the collusion of Mr. and Mrs. W. victimizing the oldest child. When the marriage was dissolved, the transference process

[7]Norman W. Bell and Ezra F. Vogel, *A Modern Introduction to the Family,* New York, The Free Press, 1968, p. 416.

[8]Nathan W. Ackerman, *Treating the Troubled Family,* New York, Basic Books, Inc., 1966, p. 78.

was assumed by the two remaining adolescents living at home, again directed toward Linda. The situation is further complicated by the scapegoating now, involving a network of collusion; the father is allied with the two younger children. All three are united in scapegoating the "identified patient." They perceive her as a dangerous force and act as if she must either be controlled or eliminated if the family is to survive.

Therapist: Give me an example of disagreement between you and Linda.

Debbie: I tell her if you won't do the dishes and stop getting on my nerves, then pack up and go.

Therapist: You say you lose your temper over 'dumb things,' Richard. Can you give me an example?

Richard: When Linda runs an ironing board over my feet I get mad and tell her to get out.

Therapist: Mr. W., you gave Linda a car and she paid for it. Now you say you had a warrant made out for her arrest?

Mr. W.: Yes, I heard she was planning to leave town. I told her, "Stay in town or bring the car back."

"The designated patient half-willingly accepts her role as the scapegoat and sacrifices her autonomy in order to fill in gaps and voids in the family relationship."[9]

"If the problem child is to be a satisfactory scapegoat he must carry out his assigned role. The problem behavior must be reinforced strongly enough so that it will continue in spite of the hostility and anxiety it produces in the child."[10] This balance of power is possible only because the parents have superior sanctions over the child in terms of what he can and cannot do. This balance depends largely on the amount of inconsistencies by the parents in handling the child. The most common inconsistencies are in role expectations and discipline affecting relationships in the family.

Therapist: How did Linda react when Debbie was born?

Mr. W.: There was extreme jealousy. She would throw a toy into the crib with enough force to hurt the baby. Her mother would slap her. I would hold her on my lap and comfort her. I expected her to act that way.

Therapist: Did you and your ex-wife discuss Linda's dating?

Mr. W.: We never reached an agreement. Neither one would make a commitment. Linda played one against the other.

[9]Ivan Boszormenyi-Nagy and James L. Framo, *Intensive Family Therapy*, New York, Harper & Row, 1965, p. 152.

[10]Norman W. Bell and Ezra F. Vogel, *A Modern Introduction to the Family*, New York, The Free Press, 1968, p. 420.

By one parent encouraging one type of behavior and the other parent another, the child is caught in a conflict. Mrs. W. incorporated Linda into her schemes to carry stolen goods from a store. Mr. W. wanted Linda to help convict his ex-wife of stealing by giving testimony. Again Linda was the pawn in their marital struggle. The conflicting expectations existed for a long period of time and Linda internalized them. All three involved people had complementary role expectations, and the assigned roles, where accomplished, were appropriately rewarded. By the time Linda appeared at the mental health clinic seeking help, this vicious cycle was a well-established part of her family system. Labeling Linda "the patient" gives stability to the family's transactional mode and prevents scapegoating from passing from one child to another.

When scapegoating has become an established pattern within a family system, a relatively stable equilibrium of the family is achieved. However, there can be difficulties in maintaining this equilibrium. When Linda was identified as "the patient" by an outside agency, pressure was brought to bear upon the family. Excessive guilt felt by all family members is acted upon with new activities. Mrs. W. has remarried, she invites Linda to live with her and call the new husband "Dad." Mr. W. loudly contests to "treating all the children alike" and enumerates what he buys each one. Debbie accompanies Linda to the park to feed ducks; that's her bargaining gesture to demonstrate she accepts Linda, and Richard spends long hours with Linda talking out her problems. All these attempts by the family to rationalize their behavior is defensive. Much energy is devoted to an "armed truce" but the constant danger of explosion is ever present. Linda's behavior is a series of distress signals that the family system is being threatened.

The function of scapegoating minimized and controlled the parental conflicts while maintaining the solidarity of this family system. When the sexual problems of this couple could not be contained within the system, the marriage was dissolved but the pattern of scapegoating remained. Linda still served the needs of the remaining family members. Scapegoating is still effective in controlling the major source of the family tensions. However, Linda's frequent distress signals observed and felt by the family system are now creating secondary complications. The scapegoating is functional for the family as a group but dysfunctional for the emotional health of Linda and her adjustment outside the family of orientation. Linda accepts her role as the scapegoat.

Therapist: (at first session to all members) What do you perceive as being the problem in this family now?

Linda: (answering first) I am. I feel unwanted by my family.

Linda's relief behavior is to escape by running away, figuratively and literally. Her pattern of constantly changing her residence, her friends, and her job is encouraged and tolerated. On the other hand, when the "acting out" goes too far, for example, her suicide attempt, the family equilibrium is upset. A fragment or spark from the signal penetrates this family system, and one or more members begin to hurt.

Intervention through family therapy can expose the existing subsystems and explain their interrelationships to the total family system. The patterns of behavior within this family must influence all members for significant change to occur. The therapist could introduce optional concepts for this family to practice. Suggested variables are shifting of traditional roles, revision of transactional modes, redefining delegation of work roles, and alternative ways of bargaining. This family could learn to eliminate scapegoating from their life style if another value system would be substituted that provides more lasting satisfaction for each family member.

BIBLIOGRAPHY

Ackerman, Nathan W. *Treating the Troubled Family,* New York, Basic Books, Inc., 1966.

Ackerman, Nathan W. *The Psychodynamics of Family Life,* New York, Basic Books, Inc., 1958.

Bell, Norman W. and Ezra F. Vogel. *A Modern Introduction to Family Life,* New York, The Free Press, 1968.

Epstein, Nathan B. and William A. Westley. *The Silent Majority,* San Francisco, Jossey-Bass, Inc., 1969.

Boszormenyi-Nagy, Ivan and James L. Framo. *Intensive Family Therapy,* New York, Harper & Row, 1965.

Frazer, Sir James. *The Golden Bough,* New York, Macmillan Co., 1927.

16.

Scapegoating As A Signal Of Distress In The Marital Dyad

Joella H. Rand

In a three-person group, a collusion is often formed by two of the three against the third. The projective mechanism comes into play against the third party who is usually different in some way. The third party then becomes the whipping boy or scapegoat (or sick person) for the group, and the tension within the system is reduced.

The Smith family fits this pattern of using a scapegoat. The collusion was formed between the parents, Jim and Mary, against Ed, age 9. Ed was the likely scapegoat because, first of all, he was supposed to be a girl and had the audacity to be a boy. Second, he is a little different from the other four because he has been labeled by a clinic as having "some neurological problems." The neurological problems have not been specified, in fact, in some places early in the chart, there was some doubt cast as to whether there were truly neurological problems. Mary stated: "Ed couldn't sit still and cannot learn" so the school made a referral to the children's clinic." When Ed's problem was redefined this spring, a suggestion was made to the family to take part in family therapy. Mary appeared quite eager for the family to do this when contacted by this therapist. From the information passed onto the therapist a plan was made with the family to meet with the whole family for eight sessions, one-and-one-half hours twice a week for four weeks.

Boszormenyi and Nagy state that the scapegoat is different in some way from the rest of the family. Ed fits this category because he has been diagnosed as having some neurological problems. It also became evident within the first couple of sessions that the scapegoat could also have been labeled as such because of tensions between the parents. Bell and Vogel contend that "scapegoating is produced by the existence of tensions between parents which have not been resolved satisfactorily in other ways."[1]

[1]Norman Bell and Ezra Vogel, *The Family,* New York, The Free Press, 1968, p. 414.

156

During the first two sessions, the family wanted to focus on Ed as the main problem within the family. The therapist would not fall into the trap, the family was set on continuing to make Ed the scapegoat. Instead the therapist saw Ed as acting in the role of the signaler of problems within the dyad. Because of this evaluation within the first two sessions, the therapist switched the focus from the scapegoat as being the main problem of the system to the dyad as the main area to be worked with. The therapist's direction was to work first on the anxiety and frustration between the dyad. Ed's problems would then lessen or at least become manageable.

CLINICAL DATA DESCRIBING SCAPEGOATING

Boszormenyi-Nagy says: ". . . (the) scapegoating process is that someone is assigned an object role by the collusive action of several other members."[2]

Mary: We talked it over and decided on two boys and two girls with no other planning. The babies just came tumbling by. The way it happened colored our relationship about our children.
(Further on in the interview)
Ed was supposed to be a girl. When I woke up and found he was a boy, I never got over it. We already had our two boys — our quota — and he was supposed to be a girl. I never got over that.

Ackerman has observed, "indulgence is prejudicial scapegoating and acting out in which all or several members of the family may participate."[3] This is illustrated clearly in the following data:

Therapist: You have stated Ed is the problem of the family. Will some speak more to this point?

Deb: Well, with his problem — everyone in the family picks on him and everything. He is different from everyone else because of his problem.

Ed was also willing to add to the discussion about himself.

Ed: Well, I have these connectors in my head. Well, I have to go to the doctor. I have this problem and I don't know — I know I have problems of reading and I don't know anything now. Bill calls me ratty all of the time because of my problem.

[2]Ivan Boszormenyi-Nagy and James L. Framo, *Intensive Family Therapy,* New York, Harper & Row, 1965, p. 60.
[3]Nathan Ackerman, *Treating The Troubled Family,* New York, Basic Books, Inc., 1966, p. 75.

Bill, with a little coaxing, added to the discussion:

Bill: A problem in the family is Ed. The connectors in his head are wrong. If he didn't have the problem I wouldn't bug him all of the time.

Ed is the "problem child" and the identified patient of the family. He appears to accept the role willingly and to conform to the scapegoat role the parents have laid out for him. He readily talks about his problems and that Bill especially picks on him because of his problem. Mary states, "He has reading and perceptual disabilities. He has problems in school; that is why we went to . . . because of his problem with the school. He isn't really a problem here at home."

"Scapegoat" is only one of many potential family roles. "Among the specific emotional mechanisms of family living, here are some that are brought sharply into focus in clinical work. Some families, for example, centrally organize their emotional life, or a part of it, around a family troublemaker, a sick member or a family 'whipping boy,' a family idol, or a family pet — family clown. In still other families, sentiment focuses on the 'doll baby' of the family."[4]

The Smith family fits Ackerman's above description of other possible role enactments very well. The family consists of the parents — Jim, 35, and Mary, 37 — five children — Greg, 13, Bill, 12, Deb, 11, Ed, 9, and Beth, 7 — plus 13 cats, a dog, geese, chickens, ducks, pigs, and a horse.

Greg carries the role of the family troublemaker. He is in trouble at school for hitting a teacher. Referring to this problem, his mother stated. "That is his problem — I don't want anything to do with it." Debbie also adds that Greg likes to take his mother's clothes and dress up in them. Then he asks Debbie to play girls with him. Mary says she misses things out of her drawers but has not said anything to Greg. This latter seemingly deviant role is not named and not openly discussed by the family. It was mentioned only briefly in one family session.

Bill fills the role of the family clown. He comes up with little quips during the sessions. He also likes to imitate some of the actors in his speech. Mary states that, "Bill is the family clown. He is planning on going on the stage when he grows up."

Deb fills the role of the goody-goody. During the sessions she was very quick to speak about the problems of the other children in the family. Bill also says, "Deb gets all the good grades and she doesn't get yelled at like the rest of us."

Mary states, "Beth is my quiet girl. She has had the experience of all of the other four so that is what makes her so good and quiet." During the sessions Beth contributed very little and spent most of the time stroking a plastic cat, with 13 live cats in the house. Perhaps Beth is too quiet.

[4]Ibid., p. 77.

THE DYAD

Bell and Vogel contend that "scapegoating is produced by the existence of tensions between parents which have not been resolved satisfactorily in other ways. Spouses can have deep fears about their marital relationship."[5] Ed is the scapegoat and signaler of the problem with this dyad.

From the first few sessions with the whole family, clues indicated that there was trouble with the dyad. Following two sessions with the whole family, the therapist saw the dyad only for four sessions. During these sessions Mary expressed quite clearly that she was hurting. There were also some clues that Jim wasn't so comfortable as he was verbalizing at first.

Mary: I worked hard trying to keep the house clean and he comes home and finds a spot that I missed. I tried having meals on time — 5–5:30 like he wants — and then he doesn't come home and he doesn't even call. I respect him but he doesn't give it back to me. I feel like I am living in a prison.

Therapist: I hear a great deal of affect coming from Mary. What are you doing at this time, Jim?

Jim: Nothing — I am comfortable. I am a quiet, placid guy who changes to accommodate everyone else.

Mary: That is what you would like people to believe, but you don't change for others.

Therapist: How long can you stay comfortable when someone within the system is hurting?

Jim: Forever — time will change everything.

Another problem area that was brought out and explored was that Mary was acting as the household head and she wanted Jim to take that job.

Mary: I am the brains for the whole family. If Jim wants to know the taxes for 1958 — he asks me. I am supposed to have everything in my head. I tried giving up being head of the household for one-and-a-half years but he never took over. He says that he married me so that I could be his secretary.

Jim: (nods his head in agreement) I bring home the bucks and she takes care of the rest.

Another area that Mary has brought up at least once in each session is the lack of respect that she receives from her husband and from her

[5]Norman Bell and Ezra Vogel, *The Family,* New York, The Free Press, 1968, p. 414.

children. She feels that she has been a good model for the children — knocking on their doors before entering their rooms, not going into their rooms without their permission. Then, however, the children walk in on her whenever they so desire. With Jim, she tries to pick out his good points and gives him "respect" but he only looks and picks out the things that are wrong. "I don't get respect back from him." The situation that Mary finds herself in is not the one that she had bargained for in the beginning. It is very apparent that this dyad has some *quid pro quos* to formulate in order to make the whole family system run more smoothly.

CLINICAL INTERVENTION

During the first two sessions the idea that the family was a system and everyone contributed to the system was stressed. The idea that Ed was a signaler of distress somewhere within the system was emphasized. Also the idea that Ed was no different from the other four was also stressed. Everyone was to work hard at not making Ed different. He was to be treated like the others — no special treatment because of his supposedly "connectors connected wrong."

The middle four sessions focused on the dyad. If the dyad can lessen some of their frustration and new *quid pro quos* can be negotiated, then perhaps the role of scapegoat for Ed will disappear.

"Family therapy must be focused primarily on the mates as mates because their marital pain is what the Identified Patient and all other children in the family are most acutely attuned to and affected by. . . . Parents who are unhappy with each other cannot give a child a feeling that his home base is secure. . . . Nor can they be helpful models for the child of what a comfortable, rewarding male-female relationship is like."[6]

The dyad has to be uncomfortable enough to make a commitment for change. They each were asked to list five statements in the following four areas:

1. Things about wife (husband) that I want to change.
2. Things I want wife (husband) to keep as is.
3. Things about me I think I should change.
4. Things about me I should keep.

Mary supplied at least five statements in each area. Jim responded to the first three items, but could not come up with any answers for number four, even after two tries.

[6]Satir, Virginia, *Conjoint Family Therapy,* Palo Alto, Science and Behavior Books, 1967, pp. 114–115.

There is some consensus of opinion reached as to what some of the areas of change were to be worked on—"keeping the house better, hollering and screaming/bickering/nagging too much and Mary not going to bed and sleeping on the couch all night with her cloths on." One of the areas that the family was ready and willing to work on was "the bickering/nagging/hollering and screaming." One area in which there was a lot of bickering by everyone was at the supper table. The therapist monitored a supper at which the new rule was that the only time a person could open his mouth was to eat or to say something nice. If bickering started, the therapist called: "Foul"; if pleasantries occurred, the therapist tried to elicit more. The night this occurred the family gathered at the supper table at the appointed time, all except father, who apparently had to work late. The therapist says "apparently," because he did not call his wife to say that he would be late. The meal proceeded with niceties and also a lot of bickering, which was not stopped completely by the word, "Foul." Most of the bickering centered around the idea that the children felt that there was not enough to eat and they wanted more of the same or something else. The reality was that the mother had set aside, on the stove, as much food for the absent father as she had placed on the table for the children. At the end of the meal a discussion was held that made overt the hidden anger at the father. The discussion summary emphasized that change can occur when the whole system works together.

Mirages of Marriage was suggested by the therapist for the dyad to read. By reading and participating in some of the exercises that are suggested new contracts were negotiated that were more acceptable to both partners.

The dyad complained about the children not following through with assignments or having to be told several times before doing the task assigned. It was suggested by the therapist that the children were following the pattern of the dyad — Mary nags Jim to fix the back door. Jim buys the cylinder for the door but he doesn't fix it. He keeps saying, "I will fix it this weekend," and this weekend never arrives. Hence the children are following the pattern that they see the dyad presenting. If the dyad is bothered enough to be motivated, it will change so that the children will have better models to follow. The dyad has, in fact, begun to move, but they still need a third-party listener for awhile to help them to keep moving in a useful direction.

AREAS STILL NEEDING INTERVENTION

During the first session Debbie mentioned the fact that Greg dressed in female clothing and wanted to play girls with her. The family needs help in dealing with this problem. Ginott says: "To fulfill their biological destiny the boys must identify with their father."[7] Apparently in this family, Greg has perceived his mother as the head of the household and his father as the weaker of the two — hence the problem with identity and his wanting to dress in female clothing.

Follow-up with the dyad needs to be done in helping them continue to make new contracts and bargains after reading *Mirages of Marriage*. A third-party listener also needs to be involved for awhile so that Mary doesn't get the feeling that she has tried everything and there isn't anything left but utter despair and perhaps suicide as the answer.

The strengths of the family need to be reinforced. The lines of communication are open at times but can be improved even more. The children are developing and growing; there were many instances where one or another exhibited age-appropriate behavior during the sessions. Jim is working more steadily now and providing financially for the family. Mary and Jim can do things together without the children, for example, going to Colorado to look at property. They are willing to examine areas to be changed but are occasionally less than are really committed toward making the necessary changes. They need help in seeing, alternatives. They are aware that change does take time, that something magical will not happen overnight to cause change.

The Smiths do have strengths. They still need a deeper commitment to try to change the problem areas they have identified. They still need a third party to keep them on the right track toward a better-negotiated system.

[7]Ginott, Haim, *Between Parent and Child,* New York, Avon Books, 1965, p. 199.

BIBLIOGRAPHY

Ackerman, Nathan. *Treating The Troubled Family,* New York, Basic Books, 1966.

Bell, Norman and Ezra Vogel. *The Family,* New York, Free Press, 1968.

Boszormenyi-Nagy, Ivan and James L. Framo. *Intensive Family Therapy,* New York, Harper & Row, 1965.

Ginott, Haim. *Between Parent and Child,* New York, Avon Books, 1965.

Lederer, William and Don Jackson. *Mirages of Marriage,* New York, W. W. Norton & Co., 1968.

Satir, Virginia. *Conjoint Family Therapy,* New York, Science and Behavior Books, Inc., 1964.

17.

Perceptual Views of Family Members of the Identified Patient

Ruth Hunt Roberts

I. CLINICAL NURSING PROBLEM

The problems of today's family are brought sharply into focus when studying the breakdown of the healthy process. Some families, for example, organize all or a part of their emotional life around a family idol, pet, troublemaker, or sick member. Others designate for members different roles such as the family genius, the family dunce, and the family clown. Still other families focus on the pretty member or the ugly member, or the group will split its allegiances between the optimist and the pessimist.

From this, it is seen that the problems of the identified patient are numerous. The family views him as different in many ways and treats him in a manner that, both overtly and covertly, relays this message. Scapegoating and labeling are used frequently and liberally, and the role of the therapist is to bring these concepts into the awareness of the family members and give directions toward possible methods to effect a change.

II. SCAPEGOATING AND LABELING

A. SCAPEGOATING

In some families the balance of blaming works out so that no one is severely damaged emotionally. In others, however, one member is always aggrandized and another is disparaged. In disturbed families the positive factors usually do not offset the negative ones, and one or another member suffers emotional injury. When this occurs, the emotions of all family members are stirred. Each feels a mixture of guilt and fear —

first, thinking that it's better that it happened to someone else instead of him and second, feeling he made some contribution to the injury. That is followed by the fear that the same thing may happen to him.

Observations of troubled families often show that one child is made a scapegoat and becomes susceptible to a breakdown. This individual half willingly accepts the role and sacrifices his autonomy to fill in areas in the parents' lives or their marriage relationship, to conform to preconceived notions of the parents as to what he should be, or to preserve the stability of the parents' relationship. He cannot evade any of the assigned roles and is pulled toward the parents when they need him and pushed away or ignored when his own needs are perceived. While outright rejection is not usually expressed, promised love is never quite delivered or sustained.

The scapegoat selected by the members of disturbed families tends to be one of its own children as opposed to someone in the community. A child is chosen because he is in a dependent position and unable to leave the family, because his personality is flexible and can be molded to adopt his assigned role, and because the scapegoated person usually develops tensions that render him unable to perform well in important positions.

The child chosen is selected on the basis that best symbolizes the conflicts. Important considerations are his position in the sibling group, his sex, which parent he resembles, his intelligence, any physical abnormalities or previous serious physical illness, and his availability. This "selection" is essentially an unwitting process.

In the scapegoating process, someone is assigned an object role by the collusive action of other members. This process requires at least three participants to be effective. Although one person may attempt to project the role upon someone, another member is needed to validate the idea of the identity of the scapegoat. In addition, a person can be scapegoated by a collusion between his critical superego and an outside person.

When family interaction is closely studied, specific kinds of scapegoating are seen as characteristic of a given family. It is usually organized in an irrational way around special meanings that are attached to differences among the family members. Although they resemble one another and share the same way of life, some are perceived as insiders, others as outsiders, and meaning is attached to the difference in appearance, mood, attitudes, traits, strivings, and values. One side of the difference is felt to be right, the other wrong, and the latter may be perceived and reacted to as a distinct danger. The "different" member is seen as an alien who threatens the security, needs, and values of the other members. Because of this shared sense of threat, most or all of the family members form an alliance to attack the different one.

These private family prejudices may be used as individual defenses against the fear of exposure and as family defenses against perceived disruption. The individual who feels inadequate and insecure may see the different one as a direct threat. The family as a group may see the assertion of difference in one member as a menace to the unity and continuity of the family as a whole.

When a troubled family is seen in therapy, the division of the group into competing emotional alliances is obvious. Each member identifies with others in terms of what he or she wants the family to do or be. Competition wages its battle around the felt threat of these differences, leading to the patterning of specific family prejudices. Three main patterns seen are the roles of the attacker, the victim, and the healer. The attacker punishes the member seen as different and he suffers an emotional injury, thus making him vulnerable to mental breakdown. The member that takes on the role of peacemaker, healer, or protector rises to the rescue of the victim of the punishing attack. The capacity of the rescuing member to neutralize the destructive force of the assault determines the amount of immunity against breakdown offered to the scapegoat. The functional roles of attacker and healer may be filled at different times by various members of the family. Sometimes the process is carried further when the person being attacked reciprocates with a counterattack. The role of the family healer then becomes more complicated and may be filled in sequence by different members of the group.

This process may serve as a link to bring the members closer together temporarily. However, at another time it may cause just the opposite effect. The less rational the prejudice, the more likely it will lead to the alienation of the family members. Depending on the emotional condition of the family at any given time, other alternatives are, to attempt to resolve the primary prejudice and ease the scapegoating assault, or the emergence of a counterprejudice.

If a successful attempt is made to resolve the primary prejudice and the pressure toward splitting the family is reduced, the family members become a unit again. However, if this movement is blocked, a counterprejudice emerges and the healer is called into immediate action. There are other alternatives to be considered: the prejudicial attack may be shifted to another member of the family; one prejudice may be substituted for another; or the attack may be displaced to a new target outside the family.

Occasionally a member tries to avoid getting into the family conflict for his own safety. This attempt at uninvolvement usually lasts a short period of time and will either fail or end in alienation.

Therefore, it is essential to identify forms of family prejudice, the roles of the members, competing alliances, specific conflicts, and types of individual and group defenses utilized to neutralize the destructive results of scapegoating.

B. LABELING

Another concept used frequently in problem families is labeling. When labeling first occurs it merely gives a name to rule breaking. If the rule breaking becomes an issue and is not ignored or rationalized away, labeling may create a pattern of behavior to conform to the expectations of others. Eventually the deviant role will become a part of the individual's self-conception and his ability to control his own behavior may be impaired under stress, ending in episodes of compulsive behavior. This individual may feel that he has reached his "breaking point" under circumstances that an individual with a "normal" self-conception would endure.

There is a great deal of pressure on the individual to accept the deviant role as a part of his self-image. Once the label has been publicly applied it is difficult for him to return to a nondeviant role. For example, the more the individuals behavior fits the label, the more he is defined by it; but the more he is defined by it, the more he fully enters it. This suggests that the labeled deviant is rewarded for deviating and punished for attempting to return to conventional roles.

Parents tend to treat children as though they were deaf by talking about them in their presence as if they weren't there. By talking about their past and predicting their future, they create a self-fulfilling prophecy since children tend to live up to roles cast for them by their parents. Labeling is a form of "role casting."

III. CLINICAL DATA FROM FAMILY SESSIONS AND NURSING INTERVENTIONS

A. FAMILY HISTORY

The Johnston family lives in a midwestern town in an upper-lower-class neighborhood. The family was seen in various groupings for six one-and-one-half hour sessions in the family home. The house was an old one consisting of a living room, kitchen, bath, and three bedrooms. The house usually appeared neat although for three sessions the supper dishes were still on the table when the therapist arrived.

There are eight members of this family: Mr. Erick Johnston, 38; Mrs. Althea Johnston, 36; Lisa, 17; Antony, 14; Mary, 13; Nancy, 10; Sue, 6; and Ruth, 4 months.

Mrs. Johnston is the second oldest of 12 siblings. She grew up on a farm outside a small town in the southern part of the state. She completed high school and married Mr. Johnston four months later. Her mother was opposed to the marriage because of her age, however, her father approved. Since her marriage to Mr. Johnston she has always been a housewife.

Mr. Johnston is the second oldest of 8 siblings. He also grew up on a farm outside the same town but did not meet Mrs. Johnston until she was a junior in high school. Mr. Johnston completed the eighth grade in school, then had to stop to help his father on the farm. Both of his parents approved of him marrying Mrs. Johnston. A month after the marriage Mr. Johnston went into the Army for two years. Mrs. Johnston lived with his parents the first year. Then they, (the parents) bought a house for their son and daughter-in-law.

When Mr. Johnston returned from the Army he and Mrs. Johnston continued to live in town though Mr. Johnston was helping his father with the farm. They continued this arrangement for eight years. Then they moved to the farm for three years because Mr. Johnston's father was ill and unable to do any work. After Mr. Johnston's father expired he continued to farm but eventually gave it up because it wasn't financially profitable. After moving back to town, Mr. Johnston worked in the mines for a year and a half but didn't like it, so he decided to look for a job as a machine operator since he had gotten experience in this area while in the service. He was unable to find a job locally so he decided to go to another state and look. After obtaining a job he returned home to get his family. At that time the couple had five children.

They moved to their new home and Mr. Johnston did construction work for approximately six months. Then, because inclement weather kept him from working frequently, he applied for and got an on-the-job-training position as a machine operator. They lived in the state for approximately one year then decided to move back to the state of their former residence but in a different town. Their reason for moving was given as an inability to find adequate housing that wasn't too expensive, plus the fact that Mrs. Johnston was pregnant with their sixth child and the inadequate housing made it "hard on her." In addition, both of their mothers were widowed and getting old and they felt they should be closer to them.

The family remained in that town for six weeks. Mr. Johnston was again working in the mines but looking for a job as a machine operator in a nearby larger town on his days off. When he found a job they moved to that town and have been there since then — eight months.

The family was referred to the therapist through a local agency because Lisa, the identified patient, was reportedly taking things from relatives and stores (six-years duration), expressed feelings of fear of dying, exhibited passive-aggressive behavior and "slow" behavior, and was obese. The agency had been seeing members of this family for two months.

B. FIRST FAMILY SESSION

During the first session all family members were present and identified the problem as:

Mrs. J.: We started having a problem with Lisa over there. She started taking things from peoples' homes. We did what we could at home. We started telling her that it wasn't right, punishing her, and depriving her of a few things now and then. It didn't do any good, then we took her to the clinic.

Therapist: (questions interspersed at intervals)
Tell about the first time from the beginning.
Punish her how?
What did you deprive her of?
What did you expect the clinic to do?

Mr. J.: I think it started in 1962. The first thing she took was my youngest sister's watch. The last things she took were some things from a store at the shopping center. But why she does it, I don't know.

Therapist: When she took something what did you say, do, immediately? (Get all the *facts* concerning incidents.)

Antony: I think that since she was a baby she was spoiled since she was the first child and the first grandchild. Now that we're here she can't have things like then so she takes them.

Therapist: First children take things?

Sue: I don't think she should do it because it's stealing.

Ruth: I don't do it because it's not right.

Mary: Teenagers now shoplift but they do it for the fun of it. I don't think she can help it.

Therapist: (questions interspersed at intervals addressed to family generally.)
What are your clues?
How was that decided?
How did you come to that conclusion?

Lisa: I don't know why I do it. When I do it I don't feel anything, I just do it.

Therapist: Do what?
Give an example.

It is very important during the first session when a systems analysis framework is used, to start emphasizing to the family the fact that the family is a unit and that no one member is to blame for what has happened. It is also important to start orienting them to telling about incidents in the sequence they occurred and to give as many *facts* as possible, that is, how family members found out about the incidents, what each one knows about them, other significant things that were happening to the family at the time of each occurrence.

C. SESSION WITH PARENTAL DYAD

During the beginning of this session, Mr. and Mrs. Johnston discussed their childhoods, how they met and decided to marry, and the reactions of their parents to the marriage. Then they discussed Lisa, pointing her out as being different from the other children.

Mr. J.: I don't talk to her as much as the other kids. I kid her and she gets mad. Sometimes I tell her that her hair is messed up or that her shoes need polishing. Maybe I'll kid her when she bakes a cake and tell her it's a little raw. She just gets mad and walks off.

Therapist: If I hear you correctly, when you talk to Lisa it's to bring attention to her behavior. What clues do you have that she was mad?

Mr. J.: She's just the opposite of the other kids. When they want something they ask for it. Lisa won't ask for anything.

Mrs. J.: She and Mary argue about makeup. Mary accuses her of taking her makeup but she won't say anything.

Therapist: What would you rather have her do?

What are the rules about privacy around here?

Mr. J.: Another thing. Lisa hardly ever goes anyplace and doesn't seem to have many friends.

Mrs. J.: Mary is just the opposite. She always wants to go someplace and I don't think she could live without her friends around her.

Therapist: You must have done some thinking about that; what are your ideas?

Have you had experience with this type of behavior before?

An attempt was made to explore their perceptions of the family members as individuals and the degree to which they saw the *difference* as a problem. The effort was to help them increase their awareness of the serial order of events and realize their competencies. Again, the emphasis was that the clinic can't change the situation but that the family has to be an active agent in analyzing the series of events that end in one member exhibiting symptoms or acting as a "signaler" of family disruption.

D. SESSION WITH SIBLINGS

At the beginning of this session each member was given a sheet of paper and a pen and told to write down what they saw as the problem. The youngest child was told to draw pictures. They were given one-half hour to do this. At the end of that time, they were told to discuss what they saw as the problem.

Lisa: I think the problem is me, taking things that don't belong to me.

Therapist: You are the signaler for the family. (to all members) It's a temptation to look at Lisa and say, "It's not us; it's her," but she is the signaler for the family.

Lisa: When I took things I didn't know why. I didn't have any feelings about it when it happened. That's why I'm trying to find out why I took them.

Therapist: The way to figure it out is to notice what happens before.

The older siblings saw Lisa as different in these ways:

Antony: One way she's different from me and Mary is, if we have money we'll spend it on something. When she has money she holds on to it. We all have about the same temper except Lisa. If you touch her she screems and shouts at you. Everybody else hits back. Lisa is real quiet. Everybody else talks. All of us are close to dad and mom except Lisa. She's more close to mom.

Mary: I like to go places and do things. Lisa hardly ever goes anyplace. Sometimes I beg her to go with me but she usually won't go. She's 17 years old and has never had a date. I just don't understand it. I work babysitting and Antony does yardwork and delivers papers. Lisa stays home and helps mom. We kid and play around with dad a lot. All of us except Lisa. I have a lot of friends and we like to do things together. Lisa never has friends over or goes anyplace with us.

Each time a family member started talking about other areas that might be a problem, they would refocus on Lisa again. The therapist must keep emphasizing that Lisa is the signaler for family problems. She may also ask how they react to that statement. A task for the family members to be assigned to do would be to list ways Lisa is like them.

IV. SUMMARY

The most difficult task the therapist has is not to be drawn into supporting the system as it exists in its present state.

The therapist generally has four choices with regard to his conduct toward existing pathways:

1. Obey the pathways, yet attempt to change the nature of the interaction channeled through them.
2. Disobey the pathways without explicitly pressing for or pointing to the possibility of different ones.
3. Disobey the pathways while explicitly requesting the use of new, counteracting pathways.
4. Eliminate the pathways.[1]

BIBLIOGRAPHY

Ackerman, Nathan W. *The Psychodynamics of Family Life*, New York, Basic Books, Inc., 1958.

Ackerman, Nathan W. *Treating the Troubled Family*, New York, Basic Books, Inc. 1966.

Bell, Norman W. and Ezra F. Vogel. *A Modern Introduction to the Family*, New York, The Free Press, 1968.

Boszormenyi-Nagy, Ivan and James L. Framo. *Intensive Family Therapy*, New York, Harper & Row, 1965.

Buss, Arnold H. *The Psychology of Aggression*, New York, Wiley, 1961.

Ginott, Haim G. *Between Parent and Teenager*, New York, The Macmillan Co., 1969.

Minuchin, Salvador, Braulio Montaluo, Bernard J. Guerney, Jr., Bernice L. Rosman, and Florence Schumer. *Families of the Slums*, New York, Basic Books, Inc., 1967.

Scheff, Thomas J. *Being Mentally Ill: A Sociological Theory*, Chicago, Aldine Publishing Co., 1966.

Storr, Anthony. *Human Aggression*, New York, Atheneum, 1968.

Tait, C. Downing, Jr. and Emory F. Hodges, Jr. *Delinquents, their Families, and the Community*, Springfield, Illinois, Charles C. Thomas, 1962.

[1]Salvador Minuchin, Braulio Montaluo, Bernard J. Guerney, Jr., Bernice L. Rosman, and Florence Schumer, *Families of the Slums*, New York, Basic Books, Inc., p. 259.

Part V
FOCUS ON CHILDREN

18.

Parental Reactions to a Visually Handicapped Child

Patricia Fitzpatrick

The mental health needs of the general public are many and varied in nature. One must realize that children are born with various physical handicaps every day. Their parents and siblings require help in adjusting to their generally unforseen arrival. Psychiatric nurses are in a particularly strategic position to meet the needs of families with handicapped children. Supervised clinical experience and educational advancement can assist nurses in expanding their roles and in functioning as family therapists. Nurses can recognize faulty adjustment patterns of families with a handicapped child and institute early intervention or, to take it a step forward, they can provide preventive therapy to help families block the development of faulty adaptational patterns that may occur when a handicapped child arrives.

PURPOSE

This selection reviews the current literature that focuses on the responses of parents to their handicapped children and to relate the theory derived from this review to the reactions of two parents as they attempt to deal with the issue of acknowledging and accepting their adolescent son and his visual handicap. The discussion is augmented by verbatim clinical examples obtained from tape recordings of family therapy sessions with the family, referred to as the T. family. Interventions directed at facilitating parental acceptance of their handicapped offspring are also discussed.

THEORETICAL CONSIDERATIONS AND CLINICAL EXAMPLES

In view of the fact that children represent physical and psychological extensions of their parents, special significance is attached to the birth of

175

a handicapped child. It has been said that a defective child confirms his parents' badness as well as their unconscious fears of unworthiness and inadequacy.[1] Vicarious satisfactions in living and the achievement of power, prestige, and wealth by their child no longer seem to be either possibilities or realities. The much hoped for "perfect" child is not, in reality, perfect and the aspirations and hopes of the parents are shattered. Moreover, the significance of a handicapped child's impact on his parents becomes even more apparent when the child is the firstborn.[2] Several reasons account for this phenomenon. To begin with, the arrival of the firstborn child and the consequent changes in role and modes of interacting are made more difficult when the child is born with or develops a handicap early in life. The firstborn offspring represents a dearer love object to the parents,[3] and the inability to love him unreservedly generates greater feelings of guilt than those felt for later-born children. For example, K. is the firstborn son in the T. family, and he developed his visual handicap at nine months. The T. family also includes two normal children and a younger sibling who is severely mentally retarded. It is clear that the parents are more accepting and tolerant of the retarded child's limitations than they are of K. and his limitations. They have had great difficulty in working through their guilt and sorrow related to their firstborn son's defect. In addition, the fact that their firstborn son is handicapped has led to anxiety about their own genetic makeup and corresponding anxiety about their ability to produce healthy children in the future. Early therapeutic intervention to assist K.'s parents in adjusting to his handicap could have prevented destructive patterns of family interaction from developing.

Every parent attempts to adapt to stress according to his or her own established defense mechanisms. In the literature, many references suggest defensive strategies utilized by parents in their struggle to decrease their anxiety and adjust to their situation. Several of these antianxiety tactics will now be discussed.

Gardner[4] acknowledges the relationship of guilt to unconscious hostility of parents toward their handicapped children. He also recognizes ambivalence as a motivational force for guilt formation but purports other psychological processes to be also at work in provoking this emotion. His theoretical formulations suggest guilt as an attempt of the parents to gain control over the calamity that has befallen them,[5] an attempt that implies

[1]H. Molony, "Parental Reactions to Mental Retardation," *Medical Journal of Australia, I,* Jan. 1971, p. 278.

[2]John G. Howells, *The Theory and Practice of Family Psychiatry,* New York, Brunner/Mazel, 1971, p. 612.

[3]Ibid, p. 613.

[4]R. A. Gardner, "The Guilt Reaction of Parents of Children with Severe Physical Disease," *American Journal of Psychiatry, 126,* November 1969, p. 636.

[5]Ibid, p. 639.

that the parents are convinced that they had the power to prevent the handicap. This acquisition of control carries the implication that they are capable of averting the recurrence of such a situation in the future and that they can cope with their role in the treatment and rehabilitation of their handicapped child here and now. In addition, guilt is viewed in the context of Kierkegaard's concept of fate as a powerful alleviator of anxiety. Kierkegaard hypothesized that the concept of fate leaves man impotent to change his environment but with guilt and its implication of personal responsibility the individual regains a degree of command over his milieu.[6] Thus, guilt can be viewed as one of the defense mechanisms of parents in handling their overwhelming anxiety associated with accepting their handicapped offspring.

Denial[7] is related to hope in that it is necessary to meet adversity, however, it often provides a great emotional distance for the parents from the stigma that their child's affliction carries and from the ramifications that a frightening diagnosis holds. In addition, denial forestalls getting involved with the problem since acknowledgement of the situation would necessitate action and change on the part of the parents. Since parents initially feel inadequate in dealing with their handicapped child as well as in working through their own feelings, they find solace in being able to deny the situation. This denial becomes pathological if it is utilized for long periods of time in order to avoid feelings of shame, guilt, grief, and depression.

The following is an illustration of how the parents of K., who is now 16 years old, attempt to continue to deny their son's handicap and their own feelings. K. is legally blind.

1. *Father:* This kid has a record a mile thick. We've been running with him since he was nine months old. He'll never get along with anybody.

K.: I need to go into a class with kids that have eye problems like me.

Father: You've had help, you were in the C. School!

K.: That school is for retards not eye trouble!

Father: If I were my father I'd fix you, what you need is a beating you'll not forget — that would take care of your trouble!

2. *Mother:* You know part of K.'s attitude is our doing. We've kept him protected so long. We don't talk, we don't see each other enough. I don't know what to do.

Therapist: You feel inadequate?

Mother: I really do, yes.

[6]S. Kierkegaard, *The Concept of Dread* (trans. 1844 by W. Louvie), Princeton, New Jersey, Princeton University Press, 1944, p. 86.
[7]H. Molony, "Parental Reactions to the Mentally Retarded," *Medical Journal of Australia, Part II, I,* April 1971, p. 914.

Father: What the hell is bugging him??! (exasperated)

Therapist: Adjusting to his visual trouble is taking its toll on the whole family.

Mother: Family? Meaning us?

Therapist: Yes.

Mother and Father: We know K. is legally blind. We know that.

Therapist: Accepting it is harder though.

Mother: We've accepted it, I don't feel guilty except that it's like what's wrong with me that I gave birth, that God punishes me so badly! . . . . I guess I do feel a little guilty especially after J. was born retarded.

Anger and blaming[8] are other devices used by parents to control their anxiety. Parents can assign blame and project their anger to society for not making provisions for their child, to the obstetrician for his faulty technique, to the family doctor for his negligence when caring for early childhood diseases, or to fate for being so unfair and cruel. If blaming and the projection of anger persists, the role that the parents must assume in successfully managing the care of their child becomes blurred. The following example from the T. family will illustrate this point.

3. *Mother:* I don't blame — or — or — or —, but Goddamn it can't they come up with some solution?!!!

Therapist: You're angry with all professionals, including me.

Mother: I really am but I know it is a complex problem.

Therapist: What part do you play in coming to a solution?

Mother: Me?

Father: We've tried everything.

Therapist: Tell me one thing you've tried.

Another defense often employed by parents in their efforts to avoid the anxiety and depression that are concomitant with accepting their handicapped offspring is withdrawal.[9] For example, K.'s parents withdrew from involvement with him as well as from one another. This was evidenced by his father taking on two full-time jobs and his mother holding one full-time job without the economic necessity for doing so. In addition, when K.'s handicap was confirmed, the family unit severed their interactions completely with the father's relatives. It seems that the concepts of shame, fear, and guilt contribute to the withdrawal response of families as

[8]P. Pinkerton, "Parental Acceptance of the Handicapped Child," *Developmental Medicine and Child Neurology, 12,* April 1970, p. 209.

[9]E. J. Anthony, "Impact of Mental and Physical Illness on Family Life," *American Journal of Psychiatry, 127,* 1970, p. 139.

they try to cope with a handicapped member and their own reactions. Mutual withdrawal is also evidenced by the fact that K.'s family members have great difficulty in talking with one another. Their ways of relating consist of silences, yelling, hitting, and teasing. They have all developed separate interests and rarely socialize as a complete family group. Hence, mutual withdrawal within families perpetuates and intensifies shame, anger, and blaming thereby making the working-through process more difficult and complex for all members.

Finally, in order to lessen their impotence in dealing with a difficult situation parents, often become too strict and overprotective of their afflicted offspring. This reaction is destructive in that it denies the child his chance to adapt realistically to his handicap and to maximize his potential for self-actualization. Overprotectiveness may also allow unconscious evasion of marital responsibilities by one or both partners. The child becomes the substitute for a satisfying marriage and gives meaning to his parent's barren relationship.[10] Furthermore, overprotectiveness can be viewed as a compensatory guilt reaction by parents for the fact that they created a defective child. This cycle of overprotectiveness can be broken if the parents are helped to take on a more natural, less anxiety-influenced approach to their handicapped child. Such an approach would decrease unhealthy overdependence of the child on his parents and also decrease sibling jealousy stemming from the extra attention and concern continually afforded to the "special" sibling.

INTERVENTION

Initial handling of parental attitudes toward their handicapped offspring can determine the degree of unnecessary doctor shopping and the potential for working through this traumatic event. Effective intervention is only possible if early, consistent, and prolonged contact is made by health workers with the parents.[10] The clinical specialist in psychiatric nursing as well as other mental health professionals hold the key to interventions that would facilitate parental acceptance of their child and his affliction.

In the early phases of adjustment, parents need help in verbalizing their concerns. This verbalization can be promoted by nonverbal acceptance of the parents' grief reaction and by a private, unhurried atmosphere in which to explore their thoughts and feelings related to having a handicapped child. False reassurances and terse responses should be avoided since they serve only to provoke anger in the parents toward professionals and to alienate the parents from the problem they must ultimately resolve. The ability to be patient and to be open to questions along with

[10]Pinkerton, p. 211.

the capacity to listen and to empathize with the parents are integral aspects of achieving an effective working relationship with parents of handicapped children.

Educating the parents is also a necessary part of therapeutic intervention by the clinical specialist. K.'s parents, for example, need to realistically acknowledge that visually handicapped children are likely to be sedentary and have a reduced working capacity in certain areas because of poor acuity.[11] In addition, there are certain vulnerable periods in the growth and development of visually handicapped children that parents must be made aware of, one crucial period being the development of object constancy. In the visually handicapped child, object constancy is slow to develop, and thus the child's need for security and need for the mothering figure to be within reach and available for touching is intensified.[12] Both parents must be tactilely oriented in order to foster the child's security and be incorporated by the child as basically loving and trusting significant others.

It has been found that very early deficiency of coenesthetic sensory experience results in gross, apparently irreversible personality disturbances.[13] If the interactions between a handicapped child and his environment are characterized by sensory deprivation it becomes increasingly difficult for a "normal" personality to develop. Therefore, parents must be helped to deal constructively with their hostile feelings as soon as possible after the birth of a defective child in order to prevent unnecessary psychological deprivation that is the usual consequence of sensory deprivation.

Group therapy, another mode of intervention, has been successfully utilized in assisting parents in adjusting to their handicapped offspring.[14] Groups composed of parents of handicapped children serve to lesson common feelings of guilt, social isolation, and confusion over disciplining. Experiences are shared and the opportunity is afforded the parents to begin to deal objectively with their situation.

To minimize nontherapeutic interactions with parents of handicapped children, the mental health professional must be acutely aware of his own reactions and feelings toward these children. Pitfalls encountered in family therapy include:

[11]C. Cumming, "Working Capacity of Deaf, and Visually and Mentally Handicapped Children," *Archives of Diseases in Childhood, 6,* August 1971, p. 493.

[12]D. Wills, "Vulnerable Periods in Blind Children," *Psychoanalytic Study of the Child, 25,* 1970, p. 466.

[13]D. A. Freedman, "Congenital and Perinatal Sensory Deprivation: Some Studies in Early Development," *American Journal of Psychiatry, 127,* May 1970, p. 1540.

[14]T. Lewin, "Mothers of Disabled Children — The Value of Weekly Group Meetings," *Developmental Medicine and Child Neurology, 127,* April 1970, p. 203.

1. Allowing denial of the situation to persist and block constructive family interaction from occurring.

2. Viewing the handicapped child as the "victim" and, by so doing, negating his responsibility and role within the family system.

3. Feeling sympathy in lieu of empathy with a resultant loss of objectivity.

In addition, it is essential that the psychiatric nurse and other mental health professionals hold the conviction that the family *can* cope effectively and that the handicapped child *can* maximize his own potential. It is reemphasized that a thorough self-investigation of one's attitudes toward handicapped children is vital if a mental health professional intends to assist parents in adjusting to their handicapped child.

SUMMARY

Parental reactions to their handicapped offspring was discussed. Theory was drawn from several sources and applied to a clinical case. It is clear that parental responses to their handicapped children are significant and demand early intervention if a healthy family system is to evolve.

BIBLIOGRAPHY

Ackerman, N., *Treating the Troubled Family,* New York, Basic Books Inc., 1966.

Anthony, E. J., "Impact of Mental and Physical Illness on Family Life," *American Journal of Psychiatry, 127,* 1970, p. 139.

Carr, Janet, "Handicapped Children-Counseling the Parents," *Developmental Medicine and Child Neurology, 12,* April 1970, p. 230.

Conant, L. H., "What Helps Mothers To Speak Out," *American Journal of Nursing, 69,* 1969, p. 2650.

Cullen, J. S., "The Effectiveness of Parental Discussion Groups," *Mental Hygiene, 52,* 1968, p. 590.

Cumming, C., "Working Capacity of Deaf, and Visually and Mentally Handicapped Children," *Archives of Diseases in Childhood, 46,* 1971, p. 490.

Freedman, D. A., "Congenital and Perinatal Sensory Deprivation: Some Studies in Early Development," *American Journal of Psychiatry, 127,* 1971, p. 1539.

Freud, S., "Mourning and Melancholia," *Collected Papers,* Vol. 4, London, Hogarth Press, 1924.

Howells, J. G., *The Theory and Practice of Family Psychiatry,* New York, Brunner/Mazel, 1971.

Gardner, R. A., "The Guilt Reaction of Parents of Children with Severe Physical Disease," *American Journal of Psychiatry, 126,* 1969, p. 636.

Johns, N., "Family Reactions To the Birth of a Child with a Congenital Abnormality," *Medical Journal of Australia 1:277,* 1971.

Kierkegaard, S., *The Concept of Dread,* trans. 1844 by W. Louvie, Princeton, New Jersey, Princeton University Press, 1944.

Lewin, T., "Mothers of Disabled Children — The Value of Weekly Group Meetings," *Developmental Medicine and Child Neurology, 12,* 1970, p. 202.

Molony, H., "Parental Reactions to Mental Retardation," *Medical Journal of Australia, I,* 1971, p. 914.

Pinkerton, P., "Parental Acceptance of the Handicapped Child," *Developmental Medicine and Child Neurology, 12,* 1970, p. 207.

Tretakoff, M., "Counseling Parents of Handicapped Children," *Mental Retardation, 7,* 1969, p. 31.

Wills, D., "Vulnerable Periods in Blind Children," *Psychoanalytic Study of the Child, 25,* 1970, p. 461.

19.

Disciplinary Practices in a Family with a History of Child Abuse

Josephine Vander Meer

This is a presentation of a study of disciplinary practices in a family with a history of child abuse. It explores interventions that would aid the family in establishing more direct and satisfying modes of communication.

A brief history of child abuse is discussed, and the family concept of "families with child-battering adults"[1] is operationally defined. Examples of clinical data from a family therapy workshop using the systems approach to family work are also presented.

HISTORY

Recorded history indicates that children have always been subjected to a wide range of physical and nonphysical abuse by parents and other caretakers. It has only been recently, however, that there has been public recognition of the problem.

The impetus for professional and public interest in the abuse of children was provided in the 1940s by observations of roentgenologists of cases of unexplained multiple fractures found in conjunction with subdural hematomas.[2]

A survey of the problem by Zalba[3] indicates that further attention was drawn to child abuse by the term "the battered child syndrome," coined by C. Henry Kempe in 1961. Zalba suggests that a more appropriate label

---

[1]Serapio Richard Zalba, "The Abused Child: I A Survey of the Problem," *Social Work,* Vol. II, No. 4, October 1966, p. 14.
[2]David G. Gil, *Violence Against Children,* Cambridge, Massachusetts, Harvard University Press, 1970, p. 2.
[3]Zalba, *op. cit.,* p. 3.

would be "families with child-battering adults" since the term "battered child syndrome" does not identify the etiological problems involved, that is, the psychosocial dynamics and problems of the parents and the family unit that result in the battering of the child.

Findings from nationwide surveys suggest that there are multidimensional factors that result in some persons going beyond a culturally sanctioned level of physical violence against children.[4] Our aim here, however, is to consider the problem from a family unit point of view. Zalba states:

The family environment plays a crucial role in the development of the child's personality, character, and social style of life. Life in an unfavorable family environment can result in a dependent, unstable, impulse-ridden, delinquent adult who will, in turn, be a poor parent, generating in this way an epidemiological chain of inadequate, destructive parenting.[5]

OPERATIONAL DEFINITION

The following list operationally defines the concept, "families with child-battering adults."

1. At least one parent has a history of being abused.

2. Parents have expectations that children will meet their needs.

3. Children fail to do that but require need meeting services.

4. There is anger at children for failure.

5. Abusive punishment is shown.

6. Battering begins to be perpetuating and children become target for marital conflict.

Data from the family sessions confirmed the steps in the operational definition. The mother had a history of being abused as a child but stated that the father did not. There was a great deal of marital conflict that resulted in divorce six years ago. Both parents had needs that were not met and took their anger out on their children who required care themselves. A clinical example relating to part of the definition is as follows:

Mother: Ah, my dad used to — my dad used to — ah — my dad used to beat me. He was a sadist. He would get rubber strips from a tube and nail them to a board and beat me. A metal ring, he got a metal ring and whipped me with that. I always wore long sleeve sweaters and long pants because — I was a mess, or he would drag me behind the car and make me run, and if I stopped running, I would fall down.

[4]Gil, *op. cit.*, p. 135.
[5]Zalba, *op. cit.*, p. 14.

Therapist: You were tied to the car?

Mother: Yes, — it was awful. I wouldn't do that. A couple of times I hit *(oldest daughter)* — with my fist. I was shocked at myself. Not in the head but — just —.

Therapist: Anger in families (interrupted) . . .

Mother: I have to calm down before I spank them. But, I'm not bad now. I beat them, yes, I know I used to beat them — like this child beating thing.

The conversation preceding this data related to disciplinary practices. After this, the mother was able to talk about some of the abusive treatment inflicted upon the children (primarily by the father) that resulted in injuries such as broken bones, cuts that needed suturing, hearing difficulties attributed to a head injury, etc. The mother was not able, however, to identify which child received what injury.

THE FAMILY AS A SYSTEM

The approach to family work used in this study is the concept of the family as a system. According to Bowen:

The family is a system in that a change in any part of the system is followed by compensatory change in other parts of the system. I prefer to think of the family as a variety of systems and subsystems. Systems function at all levels of efficiency from optimum functioning to total dysfunction and failure.[6]

If a family is hurting and needs help, an expert may be called in to provide direction and consultation. There is no blame in this approach. Identified patients are seen as signalers of distress. The overall goal of the consultant is to help family members become systems experts themselves so that readjustments can be made without the consultant if and when the system again becomes stressed.

ATTEMPT TO UNMASK

The family in this study consists of a pregnant mother, four daughters, and one son, ranging in age from 7 to 14. A male figure (father of the unborn child) was in the home for a period of eight months up until six months ago and is expected soon for the birth of the child.

[6]Murray Bowen, "The Use of Family Theory in Clinical Practice" in Jay Haley (ed.) *Changing Families,* New York, Grune and Stratton, Inc. 1971, p. 166.

The signaler of trouble within the family system was identified by the referring agency as the 14-year-old daughter. She had run away from home several times. Additional information indicated that the son and youngest child were suspected victims of child abuse.

One of the difficulties in learning about disciplinary practices in homes where child abuse is suspected is the fact that these families tend to be guarded and antagonistic.[7] Marital partners tend to protect abusive parents from disclosure as well as resist interventions by social agencies even when it is directed toward the children alone.

The first tactic of the therapist was to encourage openness and allow for ventilation of what the family saw as causing the pain and discomfort within the family system. This was accomplished by encouraging expression of what the family saw as concerns while at the same time obtaining information about families of origin.

The first two sessions consisted of family members relating many difficult and stressful past experiences. References were made to the mother being treated poorly by the children's father and other male friends, except for the current man in her life, but no information was received regarding abusive practices. Both therapist and recorder noticed, however, that one side of the youngest child's face was swollen and bruised at one of the sessions, and later marks were observed on his thighs.

The possibility of masking was considered and techniques were sought to assist in the unmasking process. Spiegel suggests "a gentle, low pressure campaign of unmasking by judicious interpretation of the undelivered messages."[8]

In considering techniques of unmasking, the therapist decided to go into the third session without consideration of previous material. The strengths seen in this family unit were emphasized, and they were told that other families having similar kinds of experiences probably would not have been able to remain cohesive. The fact that they did indicated that they cared deeply for one another.

The consultant then reoriented the family to who she was and to the purpose of the sessions. It was emphasized that the consultant was not connected with any community agency including those related to law enforcement.

A proposal was then offered to the family to work on something that they saw as being problematic in the family at this time. The mother said she would like to know the reactions of the children to the expected

[7]Elizabeth Elmer, *Children in Jeopardy*, Pittsburgh, University of Pittsburgh Press, 1967, p. 3.

[8]John Spiegel, *Transactions, The Interplay Between Individual, Family and Society*, New York, Science House, Inc., 1971, p. 130.

arrival of the newborn. The mother was primarily interested in their feelings regarding this matter. Because it was difficult for the children to do this, they were given an assignment to write this information.

The assignment worked as a type of projective technique and inferences can be made about the noted concern for the health and safety of the baby as well as family members: Feedback was given to the family about these concerns. but no additional comments were stated.

Clinical examples follow.

Son:

1. I hope the baby won't get sick.

2. I hope the baby won't get run over.

3. I hope nobody will be mean to the baby.

4. I hope my mom will treat the baby real good.

5. I hope everybody including me will treat the baby real good.

6. I think my mom will treat the baby very good.

Youngest daughter:

1. I sure hope the baby's healthy so I can do things. I hope everybody is healthy all the days of their lives.

2. I hope he's safe and that we will be safe too.

The sessions following this assignment moved more rapidly with emphasis on major problems.

A simplified version of change[9] are operationally defined in the following steps.

1. Perceptions of alternatives to reduce mismatch or to eliminate it.

2. Decision about an alternative.

3. Do it (action).

4. Feed it back to No. 1.

The task of the therapist is to move from ventilation to expectations of others to perceiving alternatives in order to reduce or eliminate the mismatch.

The following exchange is a clinical example of tactics to get at expectations.

Therapist: During the last session you talked about disciplinary practices in this household. One of these was whippings. For what can the children expect to get a whipping?

[9]Dr. Grayce Sills, conference Advanced Psychiatric Nursing Workshop, Albuquerque, New Mexico.

Mother: Cussing.

Therapist: Cussing means different things to different people. What does it mean to you?

Mother: Using God's name in vain.

Therapist: I hear you say words like hell, damn, etc., are ok?

Mother: Well, no if its disrespectful to me or to Henry.

Therapist: What do you mean by disrespectful?

Mother: I won't tolerate them saying "Go to hell" to me or Henry, or something like that.

Therapist: What other words can't they say?

Mother: The four-letter word having to do with sex. I just can't say that.

Therapist: Children, your mother says you can expect a whipping if you take God's name in vain or show disrespect to her and Henry by saying such things as "Go to hell." Certain cuss words won't be tolerated.

The mother's one tactic was physical punishment for forbidden behavior. Much of the time in the family sessions was spent in helping her to consider alternatives to behavior shaping, such as a reward structure.

Therapist: One thing I haven't heard anything about during the discussion on discipline is rewards. What happens when you do a good job or do what you are told to do?

Children: (laughing)

Youngest daughter: Popsicles!

Mother: That's fresh in their mind. Oh, bubble gum, movies, suckers, things like that. Like an allowance for poor people. The kids don't get much in rewards. I get paid once a month and they usually get something then.

Son: The other day Mom bought a package of suckers.

Second daughter: There were 24 suckers —

Son: No, 36, and Mom wrapped each one in a little sack and put them away. I don't know where they are.

Therapist: There are other kinds of rewards —

Mother: Oh — I don't know — just don't know if they understand when I say anything.

Therapist: Ask them, here they are.

Children: (smiling, shaking of heads yes and no)

Youngest daughter: When I vacuumed once, I did it twice, Mom said for once it was done right.

After more discussion about other than material rewards, which seemed to be limited, the therapist asked the children what rewards they would like for getting their work done, such as cleaning their rooms. One daughter said she would like to be able to go and visit her friend who lived about a block away. The mother wasn't quite ready for this, saying the children had only moved from the back yard to the front yard about two years ago and now were permitted to visit the neighbors on each side and across the street. The mother implied the therapist was moving too fast and she, the mother, was not prepared to consider this type of change. The consultant stated rewards are frequently more beneficial than punishment, the goal of discipline being to help the child learn acceptable modes of behavior.[10]

RECOMMENDATIONS

A therapist dealing with child abuse should recognize that this type of activity can occur in any social stratum, but is much more likely when parents lack a broad behavioral repertoire in regard to control in child rearing. Recognizing this, strategies need to be developed for the individual family — in this case, a lower income, welfare recipient with subsidy.

---

[10]Fritz Redl, *When We Deal With Children*, New York, The Free Press, 1966, p. 362.

SUMMARY

This selection presented a family system with child-battering adults. Clinical data were used to support evidence of this activity between family members. Recommendations were made to assist in correcting this deviant behavior.

BIBLIOGRAPHY

Bowen, Murray. "The Use of Family Therapy in Clinical Practice" in Jay Haley (ed.) *Changing Families,* New York, Grune and Stratton, Inc., 1971.

Elmer, Elizabeth. *Children in Jeopardy,* Pittsburgh, University of Pittsburgh Press, 1967.

Gil, David G. *Violence Against Children,* Cambridge, Massachusetts, Harvard University Press, 1970.

Redl, Fritz. *When We Deal With Children,* New York, The Free Press, 1966.

Satir, Virginia. *Conjoint Family Therapy.* Palo Alto, Science and Behavior Books, Inc., 1967.

Spiegel, John. *Transactions, The Interplay Between Individual, Family and Society,* New York, Science House, Inc., 1971.

Zalba, Serapio Richard. "The Abused Child: I A Survey of the Problem," *Social Work,* Vol. II, No. 4, October 1966.

20.

An Adolescent as a Family Scapegoat

Lois Jean Plachecki

Much is written about "understanding the adolescent." But to effect more than superficial results, to look behind the behavior patterns is in order. Behavior is caused not accidentally, and it is worthwhile to try to discover the causes and patterns both in a specific case and as a base for generating theory. When an adolescent is resentful, taking drugs, wearing his hair long, running to the "hippie colony," his behavioral message needs translation in systemic terms. Acting out deviant behavior may represent aspects of a captive object role assigned by the family system.

We are concerned with how a child in the family, the deviant child, was used as a scapegoat for the conflicts between the parents and what his function of scapegoating is for his family.

The phenomenon of scapegoating is as old as human society. Sir James Frazer, in *The Golden Bough,* cites numerous instances, reaching back to antiquity, of public scapegoats, human and otherwise. A scapegoat is a person bearing blame that belongs to others. Scapegoating is a practice designed for magical riddance of evil. It requires the existence of a group, the members of which feel threatened by some implication of evil and who agree to use an other to impersonate evil, which is ultimately to be gotten rid of through destruction of the scapegoat.

Scapegoating usually originates between the ages of six and nine when the peers push out the group members who don't "match," that is, who doesn't accept the rules of the system. There are many instances when this phenomenon also exists in a pseudopeer group — the family system.

To make the definition more functional, operationalized steps for both the peer and pseudopeer process are presented.

Verbatim examples are used to illustrate points. These were extracted from data derived from three one-and-one-half-hour family sessions.

PEER GROUP	PSEUDOPEER GROUP—FAMILY
1. A peer group with at least three participants.	1. Family of at least three participants.
2. Group codes, standards, and values for acceptable behavior of group members.	2. Family codes, standards and values for acceptable behavior of family members leading to unresolved parental conflict and severe tension.
3. Covert, unrecognized threat to the group or to individual group members.	3. Covert threats to the family collectivity and a need for tension discharge.
4. Rather than deal with the threats directly, the group focuses blame on a member who is most obviously deviant or powerless to resist group labeling.	4. Rather than directly deal with the threats causing the tension a powerless child is selected to perform this function for tension discharge.
5. Group tension decreases.	5. The scapegoat is deprived of either clarifying himself or hitting back in a reciprocal, appropriately aggressive yet acceptable and accepted manner; therefore, he is used and tension decreases.

FAMILY OF AT LEAST THREE PARTICIPANTS

The D. family consists of Mr. and Mrs. D.; Lois, 25; Roger, 22; Mark, 18 — "identified patient"; Marty, 14; and Ken, the son-in-law.
All family members were present for the family sessions.

UNRESOLVED PARENTAL CONFLICTS LEADING TO SEVERE TENSION

The therapist's premise is that Mark has become involved in tension existing between his parents that has not been satisfactorily resolved in other ways. Spouses in disturbed families have deep fears about their marital relationship and about the partner's behavior. They do not feel they can predict accurately how the other will respond to their own behavior. Yet, the other's response is of very great importance and is thought to be potentially very damaging. The partners do not feel they can deal with the situation by direct communication because this might be too dangerous. Instead they resort to manipulations of masking, evading, and the like. In general, both parents have many of the same underlying conflicts but, in relationship to each other, they feel themselves to be at opposite poles, so that one spouse acts out one side of the conflict and the other acts out the other side of the conflict. They have developed an equilibrium in which they minimized contact with each other and minimized expressions of affect, particularly hostility, that they strongly felt for each other. This made it possible for them to live with each other. This equilibrium has many difficulties, the most serious of which is the scapegoating of a child. Family data suggesting this does exist in the D. family.

DATA	NURSE INTERVENTION	RATIONALE
Mrs. D.: "Mr. D. is at work so much of the time — I have been alone with the children much of the time."	"When did his job begin to require long hours?"	To determine if and when absence became a pattern of escape.
Mark: "My father only tolerates my mother." "He is at work so much, and when he is home he reads or works in the carpenter shop. They rarely talk or do anything together."	"What are your clues?"	To determine if this conclusion is valid.
Louis: "You (parents) know so little of what the other thinks — you must not communicate much."	"How does that statement affect you Mr. D.?"	Provide parents an opportunity to verify or disagree with reasons. Parents self-esteem must be maintained or they will not return to the sessions.

NEED FOR TENSION DISCHARGE

Bell and Vogel contend that tensions produced by unresolved conflicts can be so severe that they cannot be contained without some discharge. Usually latent hostilities between the husband and wife make it very difficult to deal with problems openly between them. There is always the danger that the partner might become too angry, which would lead to severe and immediate difficulties.

DATA	NURSE INTERVENTION	RATIONALE
Mr. D.: "I don't think its worth my effort to express my opinion — Mrs. D. is *always right*. All it leads to is an argument."	"Talk about one disagreement in detail."	By describing in detail all the steps the family can determine what the problematic pattern is and then "fix it."
Mr. D.: "We have never agreed on child rearing — I was brought up in a strict home and believe children should have a chance to experiment. Mrs. D. does not agree. With the older two I went along with Mrs. D. because she was with them so much."	"Talk about another similar disagreement."	Hope that the parents will see that parental inconsistency leads to insecurity and confusion. It is not the "I.P." that is ill, but family dynamics that are at fault.
	"How was it different with Mark?"	

POWERLESS CHILD IS SELECTED TO PERFORM THIS FUNCTION — TENSION DISCHARGE

Since a child is relatively powerless and frustrating from infancy because of his unusual aggressiveness, activity, and inquisitiveness, it is understandable that such a child would be selected as scapegoat to perform this function. The inducted child is often identified with a parent whom he resembles. The child is seen as possessing very undesirable traits and, although the parent actually possessed the same traits, the focus of attention is the child and not the parent.

The supposition is that Mark was criticized by his mother for all the characteristics which she disliked in her husband, that she was unable to criticize her husband directly for these characteristics. She channeled all her feelings, especially anxiety and hostility, to Mark. Mr. D., though not in agreement with his wife, cooperated in criticizing — projecting his own difficulties and problems and in dealing with them as Mark's probelms rather than as his own.

DATA	NURSE INTERVENTION	RATIONALE
Marty: "Mark is more like dad than like Mother — he is so neat and clean about everything — Mother is sloppy."	"What are other similarities?"	To determine if I.P. has incorporated father into self-system.
Lois: "Mark is very intelligent like Dad or smarter."	"What are some differences?"	To allow individual identity to come to the fore.
Mrs. D.: "He is so sensitive, stubborn, and tightlipped except when he wants his way. He is a perfectionist about everything. He likes to be alone and is satisfied with himself. I can't trust him — he takes dope — does such bad things. He has made us all suffer so much. He looks terrible with that long hair. And why does he run away?"	"How does that strike you Mark?"	Provides I.P. an opportunity to disagree. Instead, patient agrees which is indication that the "picture painting" by a bonafide other has been incorporated into his derogatory self-esteem.

SCAPEGOAT DEPRIVED OF APPROPRIATE AGGRESSIVE MODES; "BAD" BEHAVIOR MAINTAINED; VICIOUS CYCLE CONTINUES; PARENTAL TENSION DECREASED

Since the child will not be heard, he resorts to certain behavior that violates recognized social norms, for instance, adopting the "hippie" externals, taking drugs, and expressing hostility or uncooperativeness that affects the child's relationship with the so-called "social conformists." In most instances, while the parents explicitly criticize the child and at times even punish him, they support in some way, usually implicitly, the persistence of the very behavior that they criticize. The permission took various forms: failure to follow through on threats, delayed punishment, indifference to and acceptance of the symptom, or considerable secondary gratification offered to the child because of his symptoms. While the parents had internalized social norms sufficiently to refrain from violating the norms themselves, they encouraged their child for acting out their own (in this case, Mr. D.'s) repressed wishes.

For the parents, scapegoating serves as a personality-stabilizing process. While the parents do have serious internal conflicts, projecting these difficulties onto the children served to minimize and control them. Thus, in spite of their personality difficulties, the parents are able to live up to their committment to the wider society.

	DATA	NURSE INTERVENTION	RATIONALE
Mrs. D.:	"I can't trust Mark — *never could* — he won't take responsibility for himself. He does such terrible things."	1. "Give me some examples." 2. "When did you first doubt Mark's trustworthyness?"	1. To verify if what I.P. did was really terrible. 2. Since the self-system is derived by the incorporation of repeated, significant others appraisals, it is necessary to know when the I.P. began hearing these negative things about self. Once the appraisal is accepted then the person begins to act out the picture he has of himself.
Lois:	"How come Daddy and you get together on disciplining us but never agreed when it came to Mark?"	None needed Parents responded and explored reasons.	

There are several hopeful outcomes of the family therapy sessions:

1. Presenting the family system with *alternatives of choice* — to look at the family dynamics or continue to see *one* person as ill.

2. Getting commitment to change — the entire family is experiencing pain so why not hurt usefully.

3. Examining child-rearing practices both in the family of origin of each parent and the present family.

4. Redefining "old" family patterns so that gratification is extinct.

Possible outcomes of the D. family sessions are:

1. As scapegoating of Mark decreases, serious dissatisfaction between the parents may become overt and cause a temporary parent separation.

2. To maintain relative stability and solidarity after Mark decreases attachment to the home, the next most appropriate child, Marty, may be used in the scapegoat role.

The primary goal of Mark's individual therapy sessions is to change his self-system into a worthwhile individual by developing his self-concept.

In this particular family it seems that conflicting expectations existed over a long period of time, with the not-surprising result of Mark internalizing these conflicts. When he responded to his parents' implicit wishes and acted in a somewhat disturbed manner, he could be treated as if he really were a problem. Mark did respond to these expectations, and the cycle was in motion and gained momentum. From the data obtained it is difficult to know just when Mark began to be treated as a problem and at what point he actually did have internalized conflicts since this process evolves over a period of time. It is the process of developing patterns that should be disrupted during the therapy sessions.

BIBLIOGRAPHY

Bell, Norman and Ezra Vogel. *A Modern Introduction to the Family,* Illinois, The Free Press of Glencoe, 1960.

Boszormenyi-Nagy, Ivan and James Framo. *Intensive Family Therapy,* Harper & Row Publishers, 1965.

Erickson, Erik. *Insight and Responsibility,* New York. W. W. Norton & Company, Inc., 1964.

Satir, Virginia. *Conjoint Family Therapy,* Palo Alto, Science and Behavior Books, Inc., 1964.

Sullivan, Harry S. *Clinical Studies in Psychiatry,* New York, W. W. Norton & Company, 1956.

Part VI
PROBLEMATIC FAMILY PATTERNS

21.

The Double Bind: Therapeutic Interventions

Mary Jane Carter

Larry, a 14-year-old boy has been hospitalized with the diagnosis of sociopath, adolescent reaction, and anxiety neurosis. His symptoms include anxiety and acting-out episodes.

This patient's difficulties arise from several, sometimes overlapping, dysfunctional familial interactions. One type is the double bind. The concept of the double bind is operationalized as follows:

1. There must be at least two persons involved.

2. One of the persons repeatedly gives the other a conflicting message, either part of which may be overt or covert (e.g., mother says to daughter: "Diet! You're too fat" and buys candy for her).

3. There must be punishment or threat of punishment for disobedience.

4. The actors must be unable to escape from the situations (husband-wife, mother-child, employer-employee).

5. If the occurrence of a double bind is pointed out to the perpetrator, it is denied.

6. It must be repeated over a period of time.

7. The person giving the double-level message must be of survival significance to the recipient.

The following verbatim excerpts from therapy sessions exemplify the varieties of double binds in which Larry was caught. The statements were made to him; he referred to these several times in the course of 12 interviews, and his reporting of them was consistent. His physician says that he believes the patient's perception of the judge's statement in the third example is probably accurate.

They (parents) said: "If you're going to do what you want to do, go ahead. You have your choice of doing that or going to the D home, or going to a psychiatrist."

Here, the patient is told that he can do as he pleases, but the implication is that unless what he does pleases his parents, he will be punished.

That morning my sisters wanted to borrow my shirt — and that night my parents started yelling at me about I didn't hang up my clothes, and I told them I did, somebody must have borrowed it and then they didn't believe me, and they said "We'll talk this over when we get back from getting the brake and light sticker."

More than two persons can be engaged in a double-bind interaction. In this example, the patient is bound because either course of action he chooses — telling on his sisters or admitting that he did not hang up the shirt — will bring punishment. His sisters allow the bind to exist by not telling of their part in the interaction.

According to Boszormenyi-Nagy[1] Bateson describes a double-bind situation as one where a person is "caught up in an on-going system which produces conflicting definitions of the relationship and consequent subjective distress." This variety of bind is shown in the following example:

Really, no one has custody over me, because when my parents got a divorce they were fighting over me and then finally I went with my dad and the judge said when I turned fourteen I could live with my grandparents, or my mother, or my father, or in a foster home, so, you know, no one really has custody over me.

This places the patient in an impossible position: the interrelationships among the various family members named are such that any choice he would make would be wrong.

The patient has reacted to the dysfunctional processes operating in his family (including the double bind) by becoming very anxious and angry and by acting out — fighting, running away, sniffing glue, and smoking marijuana.

At the recommendation of his physician, Larry was sent to a boy's ranch where he is to remain for four years. The doctor planned this transfer in conference with Larry's father and stepmother and a social worker. Because of this, conjoint family therapy was not feasible at this time, although without doubt the family urgently needs therapy and will probably continue pathological patterns despite the removal of the patient from the home.

In view of the foregoing, and because family concepts cannot be applied in one-to-one interview situations, the discussion of therapeutic

---

[1]Ivan Boszormenyi-Nagy and James L. Framo, eds., *Intensive Family Therapy,* New York, Harper & Row, 1965.

intervention by the nurse is presented from two viewpoints. (1) Interventions are presented that could be employed during nurse-patient interviews and that would be useful to the patient in dealing with the *effects* of the double bind. Verbatim extracts from interview situations with Larry are presented along with comments about the interventions used. (2) Interventions that could be used in family therapy and that are designed to disrupt the double bind *itself* are listed in connection with verbatim data taken from a different family situation and from the literature.

The purposes of therapeutic intervention when accounts of double binding occur in one-to-one nurse-patient interview are:

1. To enable the patient to deal with his anxiety.

2. To enable him to recognize a double bind.

3. To enable him to connect his anxiety to the double-bind situation when that is the probable cause of the anxiety.

Examples of interventions that can be used in nurse-patient interview to enable the patient to deal with the effects of the double bind:

I. Purpose: to deal with anxiety (i.e., to observe it, identify it as such, and designate the relief behaviors; to elicit what the expectations were before the anxiety occurred and what happened instead).

The patient had previously defined "uptight" to mean nervous.

P: I'm getting up tight.	Names anxiety.
N: What do you do when you get up tight?	Nurse asks for description of relief behaviors.
P: I beat on things.	
N: Be my guest — you can't hurt me or break things, but you can beat to your heart's content.	Nurse sets limits. Nurse statement tends to reduce anxiety.
P: I'm not uptight yet — I'm only getting that way.	Patient denies anxiety.
N: What were you thinking just before you began to feel uptight?	Nurse attempts to get described the thought or event that preceded the anxiety.
P: Nothing. I was talking — and it gets me uptight because of these things that have happened to me.	Nurse's subsequent questions should have been directed toward enabling the patient to name expectations:
Patient left the area.	"What do you expect to happen when you talk to me?"
	"Say some more about talking."
	"Feeling bothered when you talk, when did that start?"

If patient does not reply to the above:

"You have a choice: talk and learn to understand what it is that gets you bothered, or don't talk, and go on being bothered."

II. Purpose: to enable the patient to recognize the double bind, and to introduce to him the possibility of asking for clarification.

P: They said: "If you're going to do what you want to do, go ahead. You have your choice of doing that or going to the D. home, or going to a psychiatrist."

(Despite their separation on this page, the interchanges quoted at left followed in direct sequence.)

N: What happened then?

Nonpertinent and not useful in this context; a better statement or question would have been:

"What did you think your dad meant?"
"What was your reaction to that?"
"What did that statement mean to you?"
"How did you interpret that?'

P: Nothing. I just sat there.

N.: Did you ask your dad to explain about that?

An attempt to call to the patient's notice the possibility of asking for clarification. Other statements that could be used:

"What your dad said seems to me to have several parts. Did you ask him about that?"

"Did you talk to your dad about what he meant when he said 'If you're going to do what you want to do, go ahead.'?"

P.: No, man, you don't ask my dad questions.

III. Purpose: to discover if the patient felt anxiety at the time of the incident quoted above and, if so, to enable him to connect the incident and the anxiety with his expectations. The dialogue continues from the last quote in the same context.

N: What did you feel when that discussion was going on?

An attempt to get the anxiety named.

P: I was uptight.

N: What else went on?

That question does nothing to connect the anxiety to the expectations. Nurse should have said "What did you do to relieve that" (to get relief behavior) and *then* "What did you expect to happen?", "What did you think would happen?", followed by "What really did happen?"

Examples of interventions that can be used in family therapy interviews to disrupt the process of the double bind.

IV. Purpose: to disrupt the double bind by calling attention to it, and by enabling the patient to ask clear, direct questions. (The asking of clear, direct questions by the therapist is essential in all phases of therapy; any unclear statement made by a patient should be clarified until both nurse and patient know what is meant, regardless of a connection with the double bind.)

Husband: Louise forgave me for my indiscretion.

Wife (Louise, nods in assent)

The exchange at left took place in context with a long description and was not questioned or commented upon by the therapist, who should have intervened, saying to the wife:

Later in the same interview:

Wife: I still have the letter, but I don't think you would want to read it.

Wife is referring to a letter written to her in 1954 by her husband's mistress, who was involved in husband's indiscretion.

"But I understood when you nodded that you had forgiven him."
"Why save the letter?"
"What went on with you, that you saved the letter?"
"What purpose did saving the letter serve for you?"

Or saying to the husband:

"You said Louise forgave you."
"How do you explain her saving the letter?"
"What are your thoughts about her saving the letter?"

Or saying to both:

"Talk about the saving the letter."
"Say to each other what you think about the saving the letter, when the incident was forgiven."

The below verbatim is quoted from Satir.[2]

D (to mother): May I go to school?

Mother (to daughter): When I was a little girl, I never had an education.

Therapist (to mother): Now your daughter asked if she could go to school and I'm wondering if she got an answer from you. Should she go to school, or shouldn't she?   Clear, direct, useful statement.

The dynamics of destruction of a double bind should include (1) noticing it, (2) clarifying it, and (3) eliciting instances of its occurrence in the childhood of the parents, and (4) learning how to make statements and requests that are direct, simple, clear, and congruent on both verbal and nonverbal levels. The parents become involved in a double bind in their childhood and that behavior becomes a habit of which they probably are not aware and which their children quickly learn from them.

Double binding can be prevented by teaching parents ways to communicate clearly and congruently and by teaching them the importance of an "open system" that permits the asking of clarifying questions.

The concept of the double bind was operationalized and discussed in the foregoing, and verbatim data was presented along with examples of therapeutic interventions. These examples were categorized as unsatisfactory or therapeutic on the basis of accomplishing the purposes of helping the patient deal with the effects of the double bind in one-to-one situations or disrupting the double bind itself in family therapy.

BIBLIOGRAPHY

Boszormenyi-Nagy, Ivan and James L. Framo, eds. *Intensive Family Therapy,* New York, Harper & Row, 1965.
Satir, Virginia. *Conjoint Family Therapy,* Palo Alto, Science and Behavior Books, Inc., 1967, p. 176.

22.

Negativity as a Major Communication Pattern In a Family

Sally E. Harris

Communication is a constant exchange of information by speech, writing, the exhibition of bodily or facial expressions, and other methods.

Faulty communication is one of the major breakdown causes in otherwise workable marriages.[1]

This statement could easily be extended to include the entire family.

The message sent is not necessarily the message received. The typical pathology of interaction is the partners' respective blindness for the actual sequence of communications, so that each of them considers his behavior only as a reaction to that of the other but is blind to the fact that his behavior is also a stimulus and a reinforcement.[2]

A number of faulty communication patterns are noted in family systems. This selection explains the negativity pattern, gives some clinical examples of this pattern, and presents nursing intervention.

The operational definition of negativity follows:

1. A makes a statement or a request in a negative manner.

2a. B must translate the positive inference to understand it.

2b. B denies or rejects the statement either verbally or nonverbally.

3a. B may be successful in understanding the intent. (This seldom occurs.)

3b. A and B become frustrated.

4. Negativity becomes integrated into the family system as a pattern of communication. A tells B negative statements continually. B learns to

---

[1] William J. Lederer and Don D. Jackson, *The Mirages of Marriage,* New York, W. W. Norton & Company, 1968, pp. 99–100.

[2] Paul Watzlawick, *An Anthology of Human Communication,* Palo Alto, Science and Behavior Books, Inc., 1964, p. 5.

respond with similar statements. Focus then is on the forbidden, disapproved, or blamed, and growth is stymied.[3]

Data from family therapy sessions follow to illustrate negativity in an integrated family pattern.

The T. family consists of three persons.

1. Mr. T. a retired serviceman, 40-years-old, has lost two jobs in the past year and is now attending a technical school.

2. Mrs. T. 39-years-old, has multiple physical complaints. Mrs. T. was identified as the patient by the mental health center where a diagnosis of situational depressive reaction was made.

3. Don T., the only child, age 9½, reacts to the upset in the family system with episodes of falling on the floor and rolling and with unreceptiveness.

Mrs. T. (to Don): The reason I'm trying to get you to do your arithmetic, Don, is that if you *don't* do it, you *won't* pass and the teacher will give you a zero.

Mr. T. (simultaneously): "You *won't* pass."

Don crosses his arms as if in resolution not to do the arithmetic, frowns, and cries.

The following day when Mrs. T. got out the arithmetic cards, Don began rollong on the floor and refused to stdy. Mrs. T. became frustrated and told Mr. T. who also became frustrated.

Step IV — "Negativity" becomes integrated into the family system as a pattern of communication. A tells B "negatives" continually. B learns to respond with similar negatives. Focus is then on the forbidden, disapproved, blame, and growth is stymied.

At the next therapy session, both Mr. and Mrs. T. blamed Don for not doing his arithmetic. The pattern was repeated.

Here are some examples of how much this pattern of communication has become integrated into the T. family.

1. When the nurse confronted Mrs. T. with the number of negative expressions she was using, she replied, "But that's the way I think."

2. Don says "Don't" to the cat.

3. Mr. and Mrs. T. brought out the fact that negativity is a pattern of communication in both their families of origin.

Watzlawick says,

Human Communication is a multi-level phenomenon. First there is the content, its information value. Second, there is an aspect which defines

[3]University of New Mexico, Conference with Grayce Sills, Ph.D., July, 1970.

what the message is about *and how the receiver conceives of his* relationship *with the sender. This is the meta-communication or communication about the communication. Meta communications can be conveyed verbally, non-verbally expressed by behavior, or may be implied by general or specific context in which an interaction takes place.*[4]

Consider this statement by Mrs. T. to Don concerning the way she expects him to do his arithmetic: "Don, I want you to *not* give me a hard time about your numbers. You are to *not* roll on the floor and *not* take twenty minutes to do one number."

In context all the child knows is what he is expected *not* to do. No clear guidelines are given him about what his mother *does* expect of him. She should have told him what she meant by a "hard time," the amount of time he could take to do each problem, and the position she expected him to assume physically while doing his arithmetic.

The metacommunication — what the communication is about — was extremely difficult for the child to picture. He had to attempt to translate the negative message to the positive: "How *does* mother expect me to do the arithmetic." Since this message was almost impossible for him to translate accurately, he became frustrated and reacted by falling on the floor. He possibly thought that Mrs. T. actually expected a "hard time" from him since she did mention it.

When the nurse asked Don for his interpretation of the way his mother expected him to do his arithmetic, his reply was "I don't know." This is a phrase used repeatedly by this child. He actually cannot know what his parents expect of him because their expectations are seldom stated positively.

Following is an example of the negativity pattern in an interchange between Mr. and Mrs. T.

Mrs. T.: Don't drive so fast.

Mr. T.: I'm *not* driving fast.

Both became frustrated and did not speak for the remainder of the drive. The command aspect of both statements was nonspecific — what speed would be acceptable to both Mr. and Mrs. T.

STRATEGIES FOR NURSING INTERVENTION

INTRODUCING OF THE FAMILY AS A SYSTEM

In summarizing the first visit, the nurse made clear to the T. family that faulty communication was the most probable cause of their difficulties.

---

[4]Watzlawick, op. cit., p. 3.

Their symptoms indicated that something was going wrong in the family. The nurse explained that the family works as a system in which each person's behavior affects every member of the family. She explained that no individual person was ever to blame when there was hurt in a family. Hurts that ensue are largely unintentional. The unclear communication needed fixing. The nurse told the family that she could not guarantee that the sessions would be painless but that they would gain new perspective.

DEFINING THE PROBLEM

The nurse asked the family to say what brought them to the mental health center. This was to have the family to define their problem. The interaction that occured during the first two sessions helped the nurse to establish that negativity was definitely one of the several faulty communication patterns in operation in the T. family system.

BRINGING THE PATTERN OF NEGATIVITY TO THE FAMILY'S AWARENESS

During the third session, the nurse pointed out to the family that each of them told the others what he did *not* expect but seldom stated expectations of the others in a clear, positive manner. When the nurse made this statement, Mrs. T. said, "But this is the way I think." Mr. T. agreed that the negativistic way of communicating was a barrier to understanding. Don listened with apparent interest but made no comment.

The nurse suggested that the family try stating expectations in a positive manner to see if this approach could be more useful to them. When the nurse pointed out the multiple number of times Mrs. T. used "not" in speaking to Don she commented, "He should understand it. I've said 'don't' to him since he was a baby." The resistance to change was evident.

At the close of the third session, the nurse asked the family to write down all the negative expressions that they used so that they would become aware of the frequency of this pattern. This assignment was begun but not completed, illustrating a second faulty pattern of communication in the T. family: incomplete transactions. Mr. T. stated that he thought they were using negative expressions less since the previous therapy session. Mrs. T. stated that the family had just stopped talking to one another as much.

The nurse observed very little change in the number of negativistic statements in the fourth interview. She continued to point out their negativity and asked the family to change the negative statements to positive ones. This task was apparently difficult for them. Don replied, "I can't." Mr. T. began breathing heavily, which he verified was a symptom of his being upset, and Mrs. T. responded with deep sighing when asked to clarify negative statements.

PROGRESS SUMMARY

There was beginning awareness by the family that "negativity" has become a pattern in the family communication system.

Mr. T. acknowledged that negative statements were barriers to understanding. Mr. T. and Don indicated that clear positive statements are easier to understand than negative statements. Mrs. T. expresses being overwhelmed by the energy needed to change an ingrained habit.

EXISTING BLOCKS TO PROGRESS AND PLANNED STRATEGY

The nurse continued to suggest to the family that each of them had within himself the potential for change. She commented on every slight positive change. The nurse continued to halt each member when negative statements were made and asked for positive clarification. After this modeling, family members can check the negative statements within their own system.

The nurse could set up a therapeutic paradox based on the following quotation from Jay Haley's *Strategies of Psychotherapy.*

Assuming that ongoing relationships between intimates can be described in terms of a cybernetic analogy — people function as "governors" in relation to each other by reacting in "error-activated" ways to each others behavior. If a wife begins to exceed a certain range of behavior, her husband reacts in such a way as to re-establish the previous range of behavior. Granting that people in ongoing relationships function as "governors" in relation to one another, and granting that it is the function of a governor to diminish change, then the first law of relationships follows: When one person indicates a change in relation to another, the other will act upon the first so as to diminish and modify that change. *Granting the functioning of this law, a therapist must* avoid *making direct requests for change and bring change about while emphasizing some other aspect of the interchange, such as the gaining of self-understanding. Yet by not asking for change the therapist will have set up a paradoxical situation: in a framework designed to bring about change, he does not ask for change. It would also follow that a reasonable therapeutic tactic would be the encouragement of symptomatic behavior. When the therapist encourages an increase in symptomatic behavior, and the patient responds so as to diminish the change he is requesting, the patient will be moving in the direction of symptomatic change.*[5]

In an alternative approach the nurse's instructions to the T. family might have been "You are to make all requests and statements to each other in a negative manner. Response to the negative statements must also be negative. This will aid you to understand yourselves and one another."

---

[5]Jay Haley, *Strategies of Psychotherapy*, New York, Grune and Stratton, 1963, pp. 188–189.

SUMMARY

This was an introductory presentation of negativity as a faulty communication pattern within a family system. Negativity was operationally defined, clinical examples of the pattern were given, and strategies of nursing intervention were described.

BIBLIOGRAPHY

Ackerman, Nathan W. *Treating the Troubled Family,* New York and London, Basic Books, Inc., 1966.

Ginott, Haim G., Ph.D. *Between Parent and Child,* New York, The McMillan Company, 1965.

Parsons, Talcott and Robert F. Bales. *Family, Socialization and Interaction Process,* The Free Press of Glencoe, 1964.

Ruesch, Jurgen, M.D. *Therapeutic Communication,* New York, W. W. Norton & Company, Inc., 1961.

Smoyak, Shirley. "Conference on the Nature of Science in Nursing. Toward Understanding Nursing Situations: A Transaction Paradigm," *Nursing Research, 18: 5,* September-October, 1969.

Toman, Walter, Ph.D. *Family Constellation: Theory and Practice of a Psychological Game,* New York, Springer Publishing Company, Inc., 1961.

23.

Obsessional Behavior Within a Family System

Loretta M. Birckhead

Salzman defined obsessive-compulsive neurosis as thoughts, feelings, and impulses that an individual cannot dispel. At the onset of psychotherapy the obsessed person does not want to eliminate his obsessional patterns — he wishes to improve and perfect them so that they will be invulnerable. It is the therapist's responsibility to highlight the destructive aspects of such patterns of behavior and next reduce their impact in the client's life.[1] Such rigid patterns of the obsessional person present particular problems for therapists when the patterns occur in numerous members of a family in family therapy.

Obsessional behavior occurring within a family system is considered here. The following topics will be included: (1) the theory of particular obsessional behavior, (2) clinical examples of such theory, and (3) intervention that the therapist uses when working with families displaying obsessional behavior with special emphasis on problems encountered by a beginning therapist. The particular examples of obsessional behavior will be presented within a family systems approach to therapy with families. A system is defined as a multilayered hierarchial organization characterized by: (1) openness, (2) wholeness, (3) information exchange, (4) feedback mechanisms, and (5) goal directedness.[2]

OPENNESS

Buckley states that when a system is open, it is not merely engaging in interchanges with the environment but that this interchange is an essential

---

[1]Leon Salzman, *The Obsessive Personality,* New York, Science House, 1968, pp. 9, 93.
[2]Fredda Herz, "For the Nurse: A Framework and Techniques for Family Therapy (unpublished paper), 1971, p. 2.

factor underlying the system's viability, its reproductive ability, and its ability to change. The environment is basic to the system in the intimate system-environment transactions that account for the particular adaptation and evolution of complex systems. The response of closed systems to an intrusion of environmental events is a loss of organization or an increase in entropy — to "run down."[3]

The K. family is not an independent system. It is continually interacting with other family systems, the local community, the school system, and numerous additional systems. The K. family constantly exchanges ideas, materials, and experiences with these other systems, and through such exchanges the family in influenced by their interactions with these other systems. The degree of openness to these other systems, and the manner in which the family system handles the exchange experienced in such openness, was definitely influenced by the obsessionalism within the K. family.

The K. family itself was referred to the community mental health center for family therapy by a child study team. Mr. K. is 33 years old; Mrs. K. is 31. They have one son, M., who is 8 and a daughter, J. A., who is 6 years old. M. was evaluated by the child study team and was found to have a neurological learning disability. J.A. appears to be functioning satisfactorily in school. Mr. K. has a doctorate in the field of science and is involved in teaching and research. Mrs. K. has a high school diploma and is not employed. The family income is approximately $16,500, and the family's home appears to be similar to those of other upper-middle-class suburban communities. Only the four members of the immediate family live in the home although both parents' extended families are in the state.

Gelfman[4] described rigidity as a personality pattern often found in obsessed individuals. Mr. K. exemplified this by his rigid interpretation of data coming into the family system. He stated: "If I give M. a pill before bedtime, I think this will lead M. to become a drug addict." Both Mr. and Mrs. K. continued in this rigid stance despite information from the therapist describing the use of Ritalin given at bedtime to children with learning disabilities and concomitant hyperactivity difficulties. In addition, the therapist worked with the family in discussing the types and amounts of medications that Mr. and Mrs. K. took, the role and attitudes concerning medications in the homes of Mr. and Mrs. K. when they were children, the importance of the understanding that M. has concerning why he takes certain pills, the incorrect connection of M.'s taking Ritalin with his becoming a drug addict, and the amount of sleep that M. gets when he

[3]Walter Buckley, *Sociology and Modern Systems Theory,* Englewood Cliffs, New Jersey, Prentice-Hall, Inc., 1967, pp. 50–51.

[4]Morris Gelfman, "The Role of Irresponsibility in Obsessive-Compulsive Neurosis," *International Journal of Psychoanalysis,* 1970, p. 44.

is hyperactive and takes Ritalin before bedtime as compared to the sleep he gets when he is hyperactive and does not take the medication. The therapist also tried to discern if there were occurrences within the family system that would cause M. to be particularly anxious before bedtime. Despite such discussions, the parents continued to be uncomfortable with giving M. Ritalin before going to sleep although they did use it more frequently as required as therapy progressed.

Mrs. K. viewed the environment as threatening at times and wanted to close the family system to environmental influence. For example, she interpreted the societal system as one with a dangerous lack of control of sexual mores. She stated: "I haven't told M. or J.A. anything about sex. He'll learn about it soon enough — there is enough of that going on in the world. Last week he came home and said a four-letter word beginning with 'f' and I slapped him for it."

Glover[5] considered the sexual problems of obsessed persons and stated that the case of adult obsessional defenses appear to be a defense against the anxieties precipitated by the onset of adult sexuality and adult conditions of life. Roth[6] also considered the sexual problems of obsessives and stressed the relation of the need for control in obsessives to their inability to express sexual impulses freely with a loss of control while maintaining confidence of success. The writer dealt with such issues by discussing with the parents their thoughts and feelings concerning discussing sex with their children, talking about the manner in which sexual information was handled in the homes of the parents and deliberating the advantages of the children being able to discuss sexual matters with their parents. The therapist offered an alternative model by being spontaneous in discussing whatever sexual material occurred in the process of the family sessions. At the close of the therapy sessions the parents did not appear to be any more willing to deal with sexual content within the family in a less rigid manner. The family sessions were terminated prematurely by the parents just as they were beginning to deal with their own interpersonal relationship in therapy. It is the writer's opinion that the parents' openness to data with sexual content coming into the family system from the environment would have become greater as the parents examined the nature of sex in their own relationship. Numerous clues indicating sexual problems between the parents were evidenced in the data of the family sessions, but the parents considered looking at their own relationship to be so threatening that this anxiety led, in part, to their terminating family therapy.

At times it appeared that Mr. and Mrs. K. selected only those inputs

[5]Edward Glover, "A Developmental Study of the Obsessional Neuroses," *The International Journal of Psychoanalysis, XVI,* April 1935, pp. 131–132, 143.
[6]Nathan Roth, "Some Observations on Obsessive-Compulsive Behavior," *American Journal of Psychotherapy, VI,* 1952, p. 9.

from the environment that would support their strivings for perfection. Salzman commented that such strivings for perfection are attempts to achieve control over one's life and are based on a compelling need to guarantee the outcome of an endeavor — which is hardly ever possible.[7] Educational standards for M. is an example of dyadic obsessionalism as seen by strivings for perfection. Jenkins has commented that overanxious neurotic parents who are educated are prone to set high standards of education for their children.[8] Both Mr. and Mrs. K. at one point paid M. a dollar for every time he received a perfect score for a spelling paper. They both interpreted to societal system as placing a high value on achievement in school and stated: "M. has got to do well in school — education is so important now." The parents insisted on an excellent performance despite the fact that such a performance would have been difficult for a child with a learning disability.

The therapist worked with such perfectionistic demands by pointing out that while M. might be behind some others in his class, it did not mean that he would not catch up with the others, especially as the recently instigated special education classes and family therapy sessions began to have an effect on the academic and social areas of M.'s functioning. The interest in M.'s education on the part of the parents was supported and encouraged, however, by helping the parents to work on ways in which they could reinforce M. for attempting to do his academic work instead of attempting the impossible goal of perfection.

Still another example of the rigid life style in the K. family is the fact that they appeared to be isolated from other systems. They only went out as a group, usually, to shop in the shopping centers. Mrs. K. resisted going with her husband on a trip because she did not want to leave the children "with just anyone, even someone from a babysitting agency." At one point, the parents commented that they each have their own schedules: Mr. K. had his daily schedule of the weekdays and nights, and Mrs. K. had her housework planned by the day. Both parents stated that they did not want to go to any activities or parties at Mr. K.'s place of work. The parents remarked that they knew no couples with whom they were friends.

The therapist worked with such isolation by examining with the family members what had happened during those times when the family did have the opportunity to venture out from the home. It was found that frequently the parents interpreted each other's behavior without verifying their hunches. Mr. K. thought that Mrs. K. did not want to go out to a movie or to some other function because she could not find a babysitter or

[7]Salzman, The Obsessive Personality, pp. 17–18.
[8]Richard L. Jenkins, "Psychiatric Syndromes in Children and Their Relation to Family Background," American Journal of Orthopsychiatry, XXXVI, April 1966, p. 455.

because she was busy with the housework. Mrs. K. stated that she thought Mr. K. did not want to go out because he never asked her to. The parents' seeming eagerness to avoid one another was brought to their attention. Mrs. K. also discussed her thoughts that Mr. K. did not ask her to social functions at the college where he works because he considered her intellectually inferior to such people. As the family therapy sessions terminated, both parents were willing to share their thoughts about moving outside their family system as well as trying evenings out by themselves. The therapist also encouraged the parents to begin to work with the school system in regard to M.'s learning disability. Mrs. K. did attend a meeting with M.'s teacher, and both parents took an interest in helping M. with his schoolwork as indicated by M.'s teachers.

WHOLENESS

It is impossible to obtain a clear picture of a family system by viewing each member separately. The family therapist must consider the family as a whole in order to understand the behavior of each member since the behavior of each member is an integral part of the whole family's behavior. The therapist should consider the nature of the relationships and the position of the members in the hierarchy of the system and not the parts of the system themselves.[9]

One characteristic of the nature of the relationships in the K. family that seems prominent is the alternation between a warring and a loving theme. Glover[10] stated that obsessional children and parents regard themselves and the family as a kind of playground for warring and loving. Family life consists of a series of encounters (such as battles or alliances) between factions, and the fortunes of war depend on how much the loving (good) parts prevail over the hating (bad) parts.

Such factions were exemplified by the K. family at the dinner table. M. at times refused to eat. His father would then become angry and send him to his room. Mrs. K. would later serve M. his dinner. Mrs. K. preferred to ignore M.'s refusal to eat at the dinner table and stated that Mr. K. was too harsh in his punishment. Mr. K. remarked that Mrs. K. did not set limits. The therapists worked with Mr. and Mrs. K. in stating the options which they had in dealing with M.'s behavior at the dinner table. After trying to come to some agreement the parents were able to concur on one tactic that they were both comfortable with. Thus, the factions of Mrs. K. and M. warring against Mr. K. was altered to Mr. and Mrs. K. working together on how to interact with their children appropriately with a sense of concern rather than fighting.

[9]Herz, op. cit., p. 3.
[10]Glover, op. cit., p. 140.

Concerning the hierarchy in the family system, Mr. K. appeared to want to assume the role of the figure in power; he continually chose to sit in a large armchair in the room rather than on the couch with the rest of the family. Also, Mr. K. remarked that Mrs. K. should read more meaningful material. He then stated, "Oh, I forgot — you can't read." To this M. stated, "I can't either I guess." Thus, both the mother and M. sensed the disappointment that Mr. K. had concerning them from his position as being the one with the education. M. did have difficulty reading because of his perceptual problem, and Mrs. K. appeared to have other values than those of her husband concerning reading, but Mr. K. interpreted such occurrences as an indication of his more powerful position. Willner[11] commented that the obsessive uses his interest and ability to support the ideal image he has of himself and to deflate others around him. Mr. K. appeared to have such an image.

In the therapy sessions Mrs. K. was encouraged to state her feelings concerning the one-down position in which she believed her husband placed her. She was also asked by the therapist to give some examples of when she thought we was not appropriately considered by her husband; she was encouraged to consider how she accepted this inferior position without confronting her husband with such occurrences. Although Mrs. K. refused to entertain the possibility of developing interests outside the home, Mr. K. did admit during one of the last sessions that he realized his wife thought she was a slave.

INFORMATION EXCHANGE

Information is communicated both verbally and nonverbally within the family. The nature of this information exchange, whether through content or process, helps to determine the nature of the relationships within the family.[12] Watzlawick and others state that there are factors intrinsic to the communication process that serve to bind and perpetuate a relationship. The manifest messages exchanged during communication become part of the particular interpersonal context and place their restrictions on additional interactions.[13]

One important characteristic of the information exchange in the K. family is that such information frequently concerned labeling M. as the one with difficulties. On numerous occasions both parents stated, "This shouldn't be a marriage therapy session, M. is the problem." On a

[11]Gerda Willner, "The Role of Anxiety in Obsessive-Compulsive Disorders," *American Journal of Psychoanalysis,* XXVIII, 1968, p. 204.

[12]Herz, op. cit., p. 3.

[13]Paul Watzlawick et al. *Pragmatics of Human Communication,* New York, W. W. Norton & Company, 1967, p. 131–132.

number of occasions when M. hesitated to speak, both parents agreed that M. should "talk to the therapist alone since he is self-conscious with the parents around." Thus, the parents appeared to consider the therapist's role as one of "fixing" M. while both Mr. and Mrs. K. sought to avoid considering the effect of their information exchange with M.

The therapist did talk with the parents and M. concerning M.'s behavior. However, the sessions did not focus around M. but around problematic patterns of information exchange. When the parents focused on M. as a way to avoid other problematic areas, the therapist interpreted this. Explaining the family systems model in which all parts of the family system are important, not just M., also helped to avoid labeling M. as the only difficulty in the family.

Another problematic area of information exchange that occurred in the K. family concerned the overstructuring of situations by the parents. Reed[14] considered such overstructuring as an obsessional trait. Such individuals have difficulty going from one brief category to another and are unable to structure information spontaneously. Thus, instead of reacting to M. in a spontaneous manner when he refused to eat dinner, the parents persistently argued about the proper discipline and their rationale for doing so. They included many details such as the number of cookies M. would get after dinner.

Another example of such overstructuring is the manner of communication used by both Mr. and Mrs. K. Both attempted to be articulate in speech and exacting in dress. They seemed rigid and inflexible in their actions. Errors were acknowledged "in passing" without appealing for compassion and with a great deal of sorting through of their thoughts before responding. When one of the marital partners did react spontaneously, the other appeared to respond not to the content of the communication but to the process of the communication. Their defenses then increased, and their communication was frequently filled with much anxiety. This was also exemplified on the parental-child level when M. asked his mother on one occasion why he was being punished. His mother then increased the punishment without responding to M. because "he was only trying to get control of me. That's why he says things like that."

The therapist dealt with overstructuring by being spontaneous and by pointing out to the parents those instances when they concentrated on the details of an experience. Comments by the therapists such as "we can get back to that if there is time, . . . what about the feelings you had at the time. . . ." Such tactics helped to preserve the self-esteem of the parents. The therapists also helped the patients to formulate techniques to deal with the behavior of the children which the parents found difficult. In this

[14]G. F. Reed, "'Under-inclusion' — A Characteristic of Obsessional Personality: II," *British Journal of Psychiatry*, CXV, 1969, pp. 787–789.

way the parents became more confident in their position as parents with a concomitant decrease in structuring of communication and greater spontaneity. As situations that had occurred within the family were examined and the intent behind the communication verified, there tended to be less of a readiness to respond to only the process level of the communication interchange.

FEEDBACK MECHANISMS

Feedback is the process in which the family members regulate the behavior of its members. Through feedback, the information between family members and other systems is handled. The family system judges information according to its goals and then acts on this judgment.[15] This judgment may indicate that corrective action is needed since the output response is outside the desired goal parameters or the goals themselves change.[16]

Salzman[17] stated that the main issue in obsessional thinking is control. The overriding purpose of the behavior is to attempt to achieve some security in an uncertain world. Such attempts to control appear to be the primary characteristic of the feedback mechanisms in the K. family. The parents frequently interpreted the behavior on the part of the children as examples of challenges to parental control. In the example of M. asking why he was being punished, Mrs. K. appeared to be threatened by what she interpreted as a challenge to her authority as a parent. In addition, the parents seemed to want to control every aspect of the lives of their children. Mr. K. remarked that "M. doesn't talk to me about his problems," and Mrs. K. worked at the same school that M. attended so that she "could keep a watch on him." Mrs. K. tried various tactics to "get the boys in the neighborhood to be friends with M."

M. also appeared to be concerned with control. The fact that M. was adopting many of the characteristics of his obsessive parents is not surprising. Rosenberg[18] described an increased incidence of obsessive personalities among the first-degree relatives of obsessive parents. Kayton and Borge stated that firstborn males are especially prone to obsessive behavior. This is due to (1) a period of concentrated exposure to adults without sibling influence, (2) greater achievement expectations of the child, especially if a male, and (3) the relative inexperience of the parents in their roles.[19]

[15]Herz, op. cit., p. 3.
[16]Buckley, op. cit., pp. 174, 176.
[17]Salzman, op. cit., p. 13.
[18]C. M. Rosenberg, "Familial Aspects of Obsessional Neurosis," *American Journal of Psychiatry*, CXIII, 1967, p. 405.
[19]Lawrence Kayton and George Borge, "Birth Order and the Obsessive-Compulsive Character," *Archives of General Psychiatry*, XVII December 1967, p. 754.

M. had numerous experiences with fire setting and, on one occasion, almost set fire to a wooded area near the K. home. Nurcombe[20] stated that such fire setting comes from a lack of internal controls and is frequently associated with a mother who lacks understanding, patience, and emotional support for her child. The child senses the rejection of him by the parent or thinks that his siblings are preferred by his parents more so than himself. The child tries to release some of his frustration by setting fires. Nurcombe also commented that fire setting occurs where the child is prematurely socialized or where the expression of sexuality or aggression is tabooed in the home by morally severe and insecure parents. Both of these situations occurred in the K. Home.

M. also expressed his aggression due to the strict controls of his parents by beating on the cat. Hellman and Blackman[21] have stated that such attacks occur since the animal is more accepted by adult figures whereas the child is not. In addition, M. appeared to develop preoccupations as a way of dealing with the attempts to control by his parents. Sullivan[22] stated that preoccupations are a way of dealing with fear-provoking situations or the threat of punishment or of avoiding or minimizing anxiety. If such preoccupations succeed in avoiding unpleasantness and are rewarded, the child is prepared to develop a pattern of obsessionalism. These preoccupations help the child to conceal his extreme vulnerability to those people around him who increase his anxiety. During the family sessions M. would frequently draw pictures and not look at the participants. Even while talking in the session, he would continue to draw with his colored pencils.

Therapeutic tactics to deal with the extensive concern with control as a predominant feedback mechanism included examining with the family those situations where they felt the threat of a loss of control. The parents were also asked what they expect would happen in a particular situation if they lost control. Understanding the parents' obsessive needs to control, the nature of the therapeutic relationship must be one where the parents are permitted to decide on matters for themselves. Although the excessive attempts to control were brought to the attention of the parents, the parents themselves decided on what measures of control they would place on themselves and their children. Regarding the obsessive tendencies in M., the therapist reacted spontaneously with him and encouraged any venting of feelings, both hostile and warm from M. during the sessions. It was pointed out during the sessions when the parents appeared to be

[20]Barry Nurcombe, "Children Who Set Fires," *The Medical Journal of Australia, XVI,* April 1964, p. 580–583.
[21]Daniel Hellman and Nathan Blackman, "Enuresis, Firesetting, and Cruelty to Animals: A Triad Predictive of Adult Crime, *"American Journal of Psychiatry, CXXII,* June 1966, p. 1434.
[22]Harry Stack Sullivan, *The Interpersonal Theory of Psychiatry,* Helen Perry and Mary Gawel, eds., New York, W. W. Norton & Company, 1953, pp. 210–211, 318–319.

trying to dampen the free expressions of their son. Still another therapeutic tactic was that the therapist tried to become more aware of obsessive traits within herself. If the therapist cannot get unlocked from the client's struggles to control because the therapist must always be in control, either the client is trapped into passive compliance and endless analysis or the client is driven away by stirring up a great deal of hostility.[23]

GOAL DIRECTEDNESS

The goals of a family are established to aid the family in achieving its socialization and caring for the family members. Such goals indicate the range of behavior that is acceptable for the family members. The determination of what is acceptable behavior is determined by those family members who have the decision-making power. Conflict may occur within the family system when the goals of one or more family members differ from those of other family members or member.[24]

The goal of the K. family appears to be one of perfection. Gelfman stated that the character traits of the obsessive (such as competence, respectability, and admiration above reproach) are designed to perpetuate the conception that the obsessive is the perfect, uniquely ideal person who is above question. Such perfectionism, however, is frequently a mask and merely allows the individual to avoid obtaining the possible since he only strives for what is impossible.

Numerous examples of such strivings for perfection can be found in the K. family. The father said that since he was out of school, things in the family were much better and all that the family needed was help with M. Mrs. K. remarked that "We have our bad days, but I am sure that all families do. Some families I know have some terrible problems." Another ingredient in the goal of perfection of the family is the quality of separateness that seemed to pervade the family system. As long as the family members were not together, then they could avoid problems they have with one another. Salzman stated that an obsessional maximizes his control over his life by limiting his committment, but at the same time he tends to minimize his satisfactions in living as well.[25] By remaining separate, the family members avoid making the committment needed for viability of the family system. Mr. K. took much time deliberating what he and Mrs. K. could do together. By going to the shopping center that was the only "entertainment" that any of the family members participated in, the members avoided entering a more intimate situation that

[23]Salzman, op. cit., p. 204.
[24]Herz, op. cit., p. 4–5.
[25]Salzman, op. cit., p. 65.

would indicate their committment to one another in sharing such experiences. Even in the evenings when Mr. K. was off from work, he would study and Mrs. K. would do some housework. The children were usually engaged in their own play.

To deal with this problem area, the therapist tried to establish a free atmosphere within the family sessions so that the family members would sense less restraint in revealing their thoughts and feelings. The parents were also guided in exploring their families of origin to determine the degree of separation between the parents and children as well as between the parents themselves. Any parallels that the therapist saw between the parental families of origin and their current family situation was brought to the parents' attention. The therapist also explored with the family whatever means the family members were comfortable with to try to get to know one another. Whenever the family members spoke about another family member to the therapist instead of talking directly to the family member or when a family member used impersonal pronouns it was pointed out.

In addition, the therapist tried to avoid presenting what could be interpreted as a negative evaluation. Scarborough[26] wrote that the crux of the difficult therapeutic situation with the obsessive lies in the atmosphere of threat and blame the client projects onto the therapist. In working with the K. family it helped in avoiding struggling against the perfectionistic goal of the parents by using indirect communication with the client that reaches a compromise between interpretations and camouflage. This aided in decreasing resistance. This, however, proved to be a difficult area for the therapist. To allow the family to come to whatever decisions were comfortable for them might indicate to the family that the therapist wasn't working. Mr. K. remarked that "We have a problem, and to every problem there is a solution." If the therapist were to take action, however, risks raising the anxiety in the family system with the possibility of premature termination.

A family with such perfectionistic goals present a special problem to the beginning family therapist who is a novice in developing his or her techniques and theories about family therapy. The writer believes that the beginning therapist who is in the initial stages of his or her development as a family therapist is especially vulnerable to entering into what Stolorow[27] termed mythic dissonance. In this situation the client has the possibility of maintaining an omnipotent stance and control of the treatment with the therapist's aspirations, essential to his personal myth concerning his

---

[26]H. E. Scarborough, "Nature of the Dialogue with the Obsessive Compulsive," *Psychotherapy: Theory, Research and Practice, III,* February 1966, p. 33.

[27]Robert Stolorow, "Mythic Consonance and Dissonance in the Vicissitudes of Transference," *American Journal of Psychoanalysis, XXX* 1970, p. 179.

healing powers, jeopardized. On the other hand, there is the possibility that the patient will submit to the therapist's interventions after which the client's highly charged personal myth of magic omnipotence and control is threatened with dissolution. The result is an early negative transference attitude on the part of the client.

The members of the family system did try to threaten the perceived competence of the therapist. The father stated that "you are very sensitive to the times that we mention the fact that you are a beginning therapist." He also remarked that "well, I can understand that your interpretations would not be correct because you are not married and you do not have any children. Your frame of reference is understandably different from ours." Mrs. K. mentioned that she and her husband had expected "an older adult from the community mental health center, a professional." The family appeared to use the fact that the therapist was a beginning clinician as a resistance tactic. A beginning therapist with any myths of his or her own healing powers and control would be especially vulnerable and doubt his or her own skills as a therapist.

The beginning family therapist who deals with such an obsessive family system should avoid justifying himself or herself. The occurrence of ruminations concerning this topic would indicate that the therapist is entering into the same obsessional pattern as the family members. The writer found that after hearing such complaints of the family, merely stating that "I am competent, or I wouldn't be doing family therapy" was sufficient to stop the ruminations. The therapist should, however, encourage the expression of feelings towards the therapist which the family members have. This would show the family a depth of feeling potential on the part of the therapist, as well as set the stage for greater spontaneity needed by the family. The beginning family therapist should also make some attempt to consider his or her own family system and individual dynamics. Then, the inexperienced clinician could have a better chance to avoid a rise of his or her anxiety when obsessional defenses in the therapist give vent to needs for control and perfection. Then the trend of obsessionals learning from obsessionals as occurred with the family generations in the K. family could be altered. The family system could then learn a different pattern of interaction.

BIBLIOGRAPHY

Buckley, Walter. *Sociology and Modern Systems Theory,* Englewood Cliffs, New Jersey, Prentice-Hall, Inc., 1967.

Freud, Anna. "Obsessional Neurosis: A Summary of Psycho-Analytic Views Presented at the Congress," *International Journal of Psycho-Analysis, XLVII,* 1966, 116–122.

Gelfman, Morris. "The Role of Irresponsibility in Obsessive-Compulsive Neurosis." *International Journal of Psychiatry,* 1970, pp. 36–47.

Glover, Edward. "A Developmental Study of the Obsessional Neuroses." *The International Journal of Psycho-Analysis, XVI* April 1935, pp. 131–144.

Grinberg, Leon. "The Relationship Between Obsessive Mechanisms and a State of Self Disturbance: Depersonalization," *International Journal Psycho-Analysis, XLVII,* 1966, pp. 177–183.

Hamilton, Vernon. "Conflict Avoidance in Obsessionals and Hysterics, and the Validity of the Concept of Dysthymia," *British Journal of Psychiatry, CIII,* July 1957, pp. 666–676.

Hellman, Daniel S. and Nathan Blackman. "Enuresis, Firesetting and Cruelty to Animals: A Triad Predictive of Adult Crime," *American Journal of Psychiatry, CXXII,* June 1966, pp. 1431–1435.

Ingram, I. M. "The Obsessional Personality and Obsessional Illness," *American Journal of Psychiatry, CXVII,* May 1961, pp. 1016–1020.

Jenkins, Richard L. "Psychiatric Syndromes in Children and Their Relation to Family Background," *American Journal of Orthopsychiatry, XXXVI,* April 1966, pp. 450–457.

Kayton, Lawrence and George Borge. "Birth Order and the Obsessive-Compulsive Character," *Archives of General Psychiatry, XVII,* December 1967, pp. 751–754.

Morgenthaler, F. "Psychodynamic Aspects of Defense with Comments on Technique in the Treatment of Obsessional Neuroses," *International Journal of Psycho-Analysis, XLVI,* 1966, pp. 203–209.

Nurcombe, Barry. "Children Who Set Fires," *The Medical Journal of Australia, XVI,* April 1964, pp. 579–584.

Reed, G. F. "Under-inclusion-A Characteristic of Obsessional Personality Disorder: II," *British Journal of Psychiatry, CXV,* 1969, pp. 787–790.

Rosenberg, C. M. "Familial Aspects of Obsessional Neurosis." *British Journal of Psychiatry, CXIII,* 1967, pp. 405–413.

Roth, Nathan. "Some Observations on Obsessive-Compulsive Behavior," *American Journal of Psychiatry, VI,* 1952, pp. 7–22.

Rubinfine, David L. "On Beating Fantasies." *International Journal of Psycho-Analysis, XLVI,* 1965, pp. 315–322.

Salzman, Leon. *The Obsessive Personality,* New York, Science House, 1968.

Scarborough, H. E. "The Nature of the Dialogue with the Obsessive Compulsive," *Psychotherapy: Theory, Research, and Practice, III,* February 1966, pp. 33–35.

Stolorow, Robert D. "Mythic Consonance and Dissonance in the Vicissitudes of Transference," *American Journal of Psychoanalysis, XXX* 1970, pp. 178–179.

Sullivan, Harry Stack. *The Interpersonal Theory of Psychiatry,* New York, W. W. Norton & Company, Inc., 1953.

Warren, W. "Some Relationships Between the Psychiatry of Children and of Adults," *Journal of Mental Science, CVI,* July 1960, pp. 815–826.

Watzlawick, Paul, Janet H. Beavin, and Don Jackson. *Pragmatics of Human Communication,* New York: W. W. Norton & Company, Inc., 1967.

Willner, Gerda. "The Role of Anxiety in Obsessive-Compulsive Disorders." *American Journal of Psychoanalysis, XXVIII,* 1968, pp. 201–211.

24.

Pathological Behavior in a Symmetrical Marital Relationship

Judith T. Maurin

A marital relationship is a system that is more than the sum of the personalities that make it up. The relationship itself influences each partner, and this influences the relationship. The nature of the marital relationship is one significant interpersonal experience that will have considerable effect in reinforcing or resisting a vulnerability to illness. "Vulnerability to illness [is] laid down in childhood, [but] the fate of this vulnerability is determined by the interpersonal experiences of later life."[1]

A crucial marital issue, as in all relationships, is defining the nature of the relationship. What kinds of behaviors are to take place in this relationship? Who is to control what takes place? And how do these decisions get communicated? This is an issue in all relationships and is expressed in communication theory as follows: all messages have a report aspect that is the information communicated — and a command aspect that is a statement about the relationship between the sender and receiver of a message.[2] For example, a husband comes home and asks his wife, "What do we have in the house for dinner? I asked Bill to come over early because we have a report to work on tonight." The husband is not only inquiring about the food in the house, but the command aspect to his communication is that, I have the right to bring someone home on short notice and expect you to arrange a meal for us.

One behavioral response to the above issue of defining the relationship has been termed symmetrical behavior — two people exchange the same type of behavior. The term symmetrical is applied to relationships between individuals in which both indicate simultaneously their wish to

[1]Nathan, Ackerman. *The Psychodynamics of Family Life*, New York, Basic Books, Inc., 1958, p. 89.

[2]Jay Haley, *Strategies of Psychotherapy*, New York, Grune and Stratton, 1963, pp. 9-10.

determine the nature of the relationship.[3] By implication they must resist all efforts or indications of the other defining the relationship. In such a relationship, a competitive pattern emerges in which each person strives to prove to himself and his partner that he is, at least, the partner's equal if not his superior.

A symmetrical marital relationship becomes a power struggle between husband and wife. This struggle finds expression in endless arguments, the topics of which are many and largely unimportant, because any given topic is not the issue. The real issue is *who* has the *right* to make the rules, to define this relationship.

As stated above, all relationships must deal with the question, how is this relationship to be defined. The struggle yields pathological behavior when the symmetry escalates, and one or both spouses attempt to control the relationship by circumscribing the other using behavior defined in some way as outside of control by either.

A symmetrical marital relationship which results in pathological behavior may be operationally defined as follows:

1. Spouse A sends a message to Spouse B in which the command aspect says, "I shall define this relationship."

2. Spouse B responds with a message whose command aspect says, "You do not have the right to determine positions in this relationship". Spouse B does not say this directly, but by:
   a. Disagreeing with the report aspect of A's statement or
   b. Refusing to acknowledge A's message.

3. B's response has threatened A's command over the relationship. Therefore, A must defend the original message to B.

4. B must defend himself against A's control and, if possible, gain control of the relationship. Therefore B maintains opposition to A's statement. The issue is deadlocked. Neither will compromise to reach a solution for each must insist upon his own way or lose control.

5. Pathological behavior emerges when one spouse circumscribes the other by following through as he had wanted, yet saying he is somehow not responsible for his behavior. (Let us say B responds in this manner.)
   a. B thus seems to have demonstrated that A cannot define the relationship, for he will do as he pleases.
   b. A seems to have demonstrated superior status in the relationship, however, because B has had to resort to irresponsible behavior to escape A's control.

[3]William J. Lederer, and Don D. Jackson, *The Mirages of Marriage,* New York, W. W. Norton & Co., Inc., 1968, p. 163.

6. A tenuous equilibrium is reached since both have resisted control, but because neither has clearly demonstrated control the struggle will again be enacted. B's pathological behavior is likely to reappear as it is the only technique he has found which will enable him to avoid A's control. This is not a truly satisfying and growth promoting resolution for either.

A symmetrical relationship as has been operationally defined can be illustrated by the R's, a lower middle class family living in the Southwest.

Interaction	Comment
The R. family was returning from a trip, and on the way home they bought five loaves of bread because it was on sale. Mr. R. states he directed his son to place all the bread in the trunk, but to leave one loaf in the car as Mr. R. may get hungry. The son, however, put all five loaves in the trunk. In response to Mr. R's above report, the following family discussion ensued.	Mr. R.'s statement of the situation. "I can have a piece of bread whenever hungry."
Mrs. R.: Well, we didn't buy the bread to eat on the way home.	Redefinition, disagrees with husband.
Nurse: How did you get involved Mrs. R.?	
Mrs. R.: Because I let him (son) go ahead and put it in the trunk. I was the one who bought the bread.	Coalition of mother and son. Wife again states her control.
Mr. R.: I didn't like the fact that he (son) went against my wishes. He did it before you (wife) had anything to say about it.	Negates wife's definition of her control.
Son: You asked Mom first to leave a loaf out.	Again, mother-son coalition whereby son negates Mr. R. for mother.
Mrs. R.: The outcome of it was he (Mr. R.) had a "fit." He got out of the car, got his loaf of bread, tore up two or three pieces, threw it at me and all over the car, called me filthy names and had one of his temper fits.	Mrs. R. gets the last word which also describes Mr. R. as incompetent.

In the example above, both husband and wife attempt to circumscribe the other's behavior by communicating through the son rather than directly with one another. Second, Mr. R. circumscribes his wife's command, follows through to his stated goal but utilizes behavior he and the family have labeled part of his illness and thus somehow out of his control. Mr. R.'s symptomatic behavior is a way of handling a relationship that is caught in a power struggle. The above example also illustrates the way other family members can be drawn into this struggle and forced to take sides.

It is apparent that symptomatic behavior is an unsuccessful solution. Its lack of success lies in the fact that the authority issue is acted out against rather than discussed and bargained, therefore, it is still an open question. Neither has won. Mrs. R. did not have her decision upheld, and although Mr. R. got the bread, he can not get credit for defining the relationship in any lasting way because of the behavior he used. "It seems to be a law of life that one must take the responsibility for one's behavior in a relationship if one is ever to receive credit for the results."[4]

In some families certain topics will chronically be selected as the vehicle by which the power struggle can be expressed. That these topics, too, are only "screen issues" for the underlying unsatisfactorily defined relationship is illustrated by the S. family.

The relationship between Mr. and Mrs. S. was frought with chronic conflict. This conflict would periodically be interrupted by Mr. S. being drunk for days, followed by a silent truce for a short time when Mr. S. went "back on the wagon," and then the cycle is repeated with the conflict gradually resuming. Although an argument could be precipitated over almost any topic, the most frequent topics had to do with how reliably each performed their tasks of daily living. For example, Mr. S. complained about the quality of Mrs. S.'s cooking and resented her taking in ironing because he felt this interferred with her completing her household duties. Mrs. S. complained that her husband wanted only to sit around the house and as a result neglected his yard work. Loud arguments resulted over how often to water the lawn, how often and what kind of fertilizer to use, and even in what direction one should proceed around the house with the water hose.

During the course of family therapy, evidence accumulated that suggested that these bitter arguments over seemingly trivial topics were a means by which each vied for control of the relationship.

Interaction	Comment
Mr. S.: See, we never discuss any problems.	Defines the situation.
Mrs. S.: We can't because you won't discuss.	"Yes, but" redefines the situation to blame husband.
Mr. S.: The reason we can't is because when I think of a way I want to do	Restates the situation to say that the wife will not have control.

[4]Haley, op. cit., p. 19.

something you come up with a different
way you want it done. If you want it
done your way why don't you do it
instead of having me do it your way.

Another exchange between Mr. and Mrs. S. demonstrates the role that
Mr. S.'s alcoholism plays in this relationship. Whereas Mrs. S. seems to
seek control of the relationship in an aggressive way, Mr. S. responds
with aggression (arguing long and loudly) but also frequently in a
passive-aggressive manner. For example:

Interaction	Comment
Mrs. S.: I think he would be completely satisfied if all he did was eat breakfast, go to the hospital if he had to, (Mr. S. was in a day treatment program) then come back and sit in that chair until it was time to eat again.	Defined the problem as Mr. S. and thus declares her right to define the problem.
Mr. S.: When you see me in this chair reading the first thing you come up with is, "Why don't you do this, why don't you do that?"	Redefined the problem, thus denying the wife's right to define the situation.
Mrs. S.: Well, I know, but if I didn't say that to you . . .	"Yes, but" implies that her first statement belongs at the end of the unfinished sentence.
Mr. S.: Let me alone!	
Mrs. S.: Day in and day out?	Her quick response says, "You cannot issue a command to me."
Mr. S.: Would you rather see me sit here or in a bar?	Gives wife a choice using symptom as threat.
Mrs. S.: I'd like to see you busy.	Ignores husband's message thereby saying he cannot determine the alternatives.

INTERVENTION

Watzlawick et al., state, "symmetrical and complementary relationship
patterns can stabilize each other, and changes from the one to the other
pattern and back again are important homeostatic mechanisms. This
entails a therapeutic implication, namely that, at least in theory, therapeutic change can be brought about very directly by the introduction of
symmetry into complementarity or vice versa during treatment."[5]
Whereas the symmetrical relationship is characterized by the need for

[5]Paul Watzlawick, Janet Beavin, and Don Jackson, *Pragmatics of Human Communication*, New York, W. W. Norton & Co., Inc., 1967, p. 110.

equality or sameness, the complementary relationship allows for a difference — dissimilar but fitted behaviors.

During the short-term family therapy the therapist actively sought to interrupt the S.'s cycle of behavior by helping them strike bargains concerning the disputed topics and then assigning the carrying out of these bargains as tasks. The tasks are to demonstrate that things can be done differently and interrupt the conflict ridden cycle. For example, Mrs. S. was not to mention the yard work to her husband, and Mr. S. was to do some work in the yard every day at a time of his chosing and decide what should be done. Mr. S. was to tell his wife what time he had to be up the next day, and Mrs. S. would make him breakfast. In addition, each was to acknowledge when the other carried through with the bargain thereby saying the other's behavior was noticed and appreciated. This would introduce complementarity into the relationship.

Both parties were able to follow through with the bargains as stated above, and the tension within the family was greatly reduced during this time. However, neither was able to acknowledge the other's cooperation on their own. Only during family therapy and then with great difficulty could either say, "I noticed, and thank you."

The symmetrical marital relationship is a conflict ridden relationship. When one member attempts to break the power struggle with circumscriptive behavior for which he denies responsibility, symptomatic behavior develops and that spouse is likely to become an identified patient.

25.

Relationship Modes and Maneuvers

Letha Lierman

In the human interactional process there are three types of relationship modes. They differ in the types of behavior exchanged and the relative status of each partner within the relationship.

The partners engaged in a symmetrical relationship exchange the same types of behavior and each considers himself as good as the other. There is a constant challenge not so much to elevate one's position but to maintain one's status. Symmetry may be operationally defined in the following manner:

1. One goal desired by two people.
2. Tactics by each to acquire the goal.
   a. Inflation of one's own capacities, skills, and knowledge.
   b. Derogation of the other person's capacities, skills, and knowledge.
3. Temporary achievement of the goal by one person.

The desired goal in a symmetrical relationship is control. Each person is indicating simultaneously his wish to determine the nature of the relationship or to have at least equal control.[1] There is a great tendency for this to escalate to "more equal" and then it becomes a game of one-upping or one-downing the other.

Much of the conflict within the marital relationship is of this nature where both spouses are attempting to increase their status and exert more control over the other. Jackson states that the status struggle in marriage is an indication of fear of inferiority.[2] He also observed a relationship between a particular type of family history and the tendency to get in symmetrical struggles. Often the spouses come from homes where one

[1]William Lederer and Don D. Jackson, *Mirages of Marriage,* New York, W. W. Norton & Co. Inc., 1968. p. 163.
[2]Ibid., p. 168.

parent was dominant and the other played a passive role while actually undermining the efforts of the dominant one.[3]

The second mode of relationship is complementarity. It is identifiable by the difference in behavioral exchange and the resultant "fit" in the definition of the relationship. One partner is in a "superior" or "one-up" position and the other partner is in a "secondary" or "one-down" position. The relationship is not imposed on either, but each behaves in a manner that provides for the behavior of the other.[4] There is a complicating factor to the complementary process, however. It has a tendency to become more progressive, just as the symmetrical relationship has a tendency to escalate. As the "one-down" partner becomes more passive or submassive, the "one-up" partner must become more dominant. The influence of this complication on the marriage relationship is discussed in more detail later.

The third mode of relationship is parallelism, which is a combination of the two other modes. There is an exchange of positions within the relationship depending on the situations encountered.

When two people are engaged in a complementary relationship, there may be attempts made by a member to question the relationship and thus redefine his position within it. Haley defines the questioning as a "maneuver" that may consist of (a) requests, commands, or suggestions that the other person does, says, thinks, or feels something and (b) comments on the other person's communicative behavior.[5] The introduction of a maneuver into the relationship by the "one-down" member is identified as a symmetrical maneuver since he is attempting to redefine his position as equal. If the maneuver is successful there may be a change to a symmetrical relation.

It is possible, however, to have a situation in which a person is allowed or forced to use a particular maneuver. This then makes it a pseudo-complementary or pseudosymmetrical maneuver.

In the process of working with one family in family therapy, a recurring pattern was observed and categorized as a complementary relationship. It was identified as a maneuver since it had a definite testing effect on the relationship. It was initiated by the "one-up" partner, however, and had the result of forcing the "one-down" partner to act. The pattern was therefore identified as a "pseudosymmetrical maneuver" and operationally defined in the following way:

1. Complementary relationship — "one-up," "one-down" positions.

[3]Ibid., p. 169.
[4]Paul Watzlawick, Janet Helmick Beavin, and Don D. Jackson, *Pragmatics of Human Communication,* New York, W. W. Norton & Co. Inc., 1967. p. 69.
[5]Jay Haley, *Strategies of Psychotherapy,* New York, Grune and Stratton, Inc., 1963, pp. 11–12.

2. Dissatisfaction in both partners regarding role positions.
3. The "one-up" partner acts outside of the relationship.
4. The "one-down" partner acts to reaffirm his down position.
5. Stabilization of the complementary relationship.

The dissatisfaction within the complementary relationship created instability within the system. The maneuver process was then seen as an attempt to bring the system back to a state of homeostasis or equilibrium. Jackson states, "if an influence upsets the balance between the associated entities, then a compensating factor is provided by the system to regain balance."[6]

In a marriage relationship, each partner tries to maintain the behavior that provides for greatest satisfaction. With both in a state of satisfaction. an emotional and psychic balance is achieved, creating a balance within the marriage system.[7]

Spiegel[8] has studied some of the conditions that lead to disequilibrium within the marriage system. In the presentation of clinical data that follows, there will be some description of influences on the family system that were likely contributing to the dissatisfaction within the marital dyad.

PRESENTATION OF CLINICAL DATA

The Allen family was seen in family therapy for a brief time by the nurse-therapist. Since it became apparent early in the sessions that the primary family system problem was the relationship between the marital dyad, they were seen as a dyad for most of the sessions. At the time of this writing, the family has been seen in six sessions.

Mrs. Allen was born in Germany and came to the United States at the age of 15. As she reflected back on those early years in this country, she saw them as very lonely and difficult times. Her efforts to overcome the cultural barriers she felt, drove her to reject the ways was of the "Old Country" and strive to adopt the new ways.

Mr. Allen, by contrast, was a native-born American of English descent. He grew up in a small Midwest town and was apparently a very quiet, passive person. He recalled his earlier years with, "all my life I was told just what it took to please — don't drink too much milk, clean the bedroom, etc." He also described the relationship with his mother as very ambivalent.

[6]Lederer and Jackson, op. cit., pp. 88–90.
[7]Ibid., p. 92.
[8]John Spiegel, "Resolution of Role Conflict Within the Family," *A Modern Introduction to the Family,* Norman W. Bell and Ezra F. Vogel, eds., Rev. Ed., New York, The Free Press, 1968, p. 394.

Mr. and Mrs. Allen began dating when she was 18 and he only 15. Shortly after this, the maneuver was used for the first time. Mrs. Allen had become dissatisfied with the relationship.

It just wasn't going the way I wanted so I started going with someone else. Right after that he waited for me in my car after work. I was so surprised. He was so direct and honest and concerned. He thought something could develop out of our relationship and he was afraid we were drifting apart. I was really moved by that. From that point on the relationship improved.

Mr. Allen's family later moved to another city since the father had a job transfer. Mrs. Allen moved to the new city to follow her future husband and to get away from her parents with whom she was having difficulty. The rather unusual tie with her family was indicated when she went back to her former home and convinced her family they should move to the new city with her.

Three years later, the maneuver was tried again with the result of a marriage proposal from Mr. Allen. At the time of the maneuver, there were many external pressures that were affecting the growing relationship. He had just completed his first year of college where he was studying engineering. His mother had recently been admitted to a psychiatric hospital and the family was in great financial difficulty. Mrs. Allen's family was giving her a great deal of pressure to get married, emphasizing her age of 22 years and disapproving of her long relationship with Mr. Allen.

Mrs. Allen went out with another man and when the two of them arrived at her home after the date, Mr. Allen was waiting for them. There was a scene where he accused the two of them of "messing around" after which she ran into the house with Mr. Allen right behind. The two recall the conversation in the house in the following way:

Mr. Allen: I remember crying and thinking, I'll never find anybody as good as you.

Mrs. Allen: That's not what you told me. You said you would never find anyone who could take care of you like I could — financially and all that. It's sort of protective.

Mr. Allen: Deep down I was feeling I wasn't good enough for anyone else. I had a pretty (bad) concept of myself. I thought you would help me improve.

Mrs. Allen: And you expected me to help you improve, to show your mother I can bring up her boy better than she did.

Two days after that incident, Mr. Allen proposed.

During the first three years of marriage Mr. Allen was going to school full time with Mrs. Allen working and supporting the family. The first pregnancy, which came very soon after the marriage, complicated their relationship as was indicated by frequent anxiety attacks in both.

Mrs. Allen: I was violently sick most of the time but I had to continue work. I expected sympathy and understanding from William (Mr. Allen) but just the opposite happened. . . . I was scared to death about the pregnancy. I kept thinking; I'm not going to have it, something will happen . . . like abort. I knew you expected to be the only little boy around.

Mr. Allen: I thought I was going to die every day for a year and a half. I felt very guilty and ran to the minister every week. I don't know how we ever made it through those first years of marriage.

With the many reactions to the pregnancy and difficult adjustment periods, the relationship itself seemed surprisingly stable. There were growing nonverbal resentments building up, however, especially in Mr. Allen.

I didn't know what you expected of me. Verbally you would say I should go to school and do well, but there was another message saying get off your (seat) and do something.
It was after Mr. Allen began working, however, that the stability of the relationship was again threatened. He had his job and was making new friends. There was growing independence and his interests were moving outside the home, and Mrs. Allen began feeling trapped. She was completely responsible for the children, handling the finances, and most of the social affairs of the family and was still working. The maneuver was again attempted.

Mrs. Allen: I felt very much like a mother. He lived in a world of his own. There was just his job and all that and all at once I wanted out.

Mr. Allen: And then one morning at the breakfast table you told me you didn't love me any more, and that you were in love with someone else.

Mrs. Allen: I just wanted your attention. I wanted you to take some interest in me.

The stabilizing effect of the maneuver was not achieved this time. Two months later Mr. Allen retaliated and had an affair of his own. His use of the same tactic made it now a "symmetrical maneuver." Mrs. Allen became "very cold and distant," and Mr. Allen experienced episodes of what sounded like panic attacks.

Mr. Allen: I thought I was going insane. Everything was all scrambled up in my head and I didn't know who I was.

Shortly after Mr. Allen's maneuver the two began seeking outside help from various sources. There was contemplation of divorce at one time, three months prior to the family therapy, but no move toward separation was made.

NURSING INTERVENTION

During the sessions there were two main types of interventions made by the nurse therapist. The first dealt with the constant arguing that occurred during the early interviews. Focus was placed on the way they avoid the real issue, bring in extraneous issues, and exchange derogatory remarks. Her main pattern for this was to emphasize his inadequacies, and his was to call her names. Portions of the tape recordings were played on two occasions after the arguing occured. The argument was then analyzed with them. In addition, some rules for fighting were given.

Rules for Fighting[9]

1. Do not evade fighting. Fights can be postponed, but not too long.
2. Do not displace fights. Fight with the one with whom you are angry.
3. Battle by appointment.
    a. Agree on the time limits for the fight.
    b. Calmly set the stage.
4. Fight about important issues, not superficial ones.
5. Agree to be truthful, direct, informed, but not crude. *No name calling allowed.*
6. A fight is a signal to "clear the air" in a family.

There was evidence that this intervention was successful, at least during the sessions. The arguing and name calling decreased considerably, and there was a striking decrease in volume of voice level between the first and the sixth sessions. They were also able to discuss very pertinent and critical problems without having them end in a fight or get side-tracked.

The second main intervention dealt with the system problem of role conflict. The maneuver, as an unsuccessful means of dealing with this conflict, was also explained. It was actually demonstrated during the therapy when Mr. Allen went out with another woman and came home to tell his wife about it. It was emphasized to the couple that they could continue dealing with the problem in that way. The choice was given to them directly. It was hoped this offer would reinforce the voluntary

[9]George R. Bach and Peter Wyden, "Marital Fighting," *The New York Times,* Jan. 26, 1969, and *Ladies Home Journal,* Jan. 1969.

aspect of their relationship. As Haley mentions, this is a major issue once the marriage contract is made.[10]

An alternative way of dealing with the problem of control was given by suggesting they share responsibility and agree on some household rules. As a first step toward this move toward parallelism, a task assignment was made. They were to agree that one person would be responsible for the planning and organizing of a family activity. The choice could be made by a flip of the coin. After the first task, the roles would be changed, and the other person would be the planner and the first person the follower. The plan was agreed upon but it is still in the evaluative stage. Mr. Allen did make a decision involving the whole family. Even though it was a minor activity plan, Mrs. Allen agreed to it and yielded to his decision.

If the sessions were to continue, the plan for continued interventions in the relationship problem would follow the Tools and Tasks Outline[11] of competition, compromise, cooperation, collaboration. It is apparent that both partners are deficit in these skills. The next actual task assignment was to plan together one thing. Some examples which were given were instances of disagreement that had come up in the family session related to discipline problems and children's chores.

[10]Jay Haley, op. cit. pp. 119–122.
[11]Helen D. Johnson, et al., "Instrument and Manual for Understanding Behavior" (unpublished master's thesis, Teachers College, Columbia University, 1951).

SUMMARY

The various modes of relationships that may operate in human interactions was contrasted. One specific testing behavior within a complementary relationship was defined and identified as a pseudosymmetrical maneuver. This pattern of behavior was used within the marital system to maintain the homeostasis. The maneuver was successful in the early usage, but became increasingly unsuccessful as the role conflict between the two partners increased. Two main nursing interventions were instituted and described. The family is at a very crucial point in their relationship, and the motivation seems directed to change to a more parallel mode.

BIBLIOGRAPHY

Bell, Norman W. and Ezra F. Vogel, eds. *A Modern Introduction to the Family,* Rev. Ed., New York, The Free Press, 1968.

Haley, Jay. *Strategies of Psychotherapy,* New York, Grune and Stratton Inc., 1963.

Johnson, Helen D., et al. "Instrument and Manual for Understanding Behavior" (unpublished master's thesis) Teachers College, Columbia University, 1951.

Lederer, William and Don D. Jackson. *Mirages of Marriage,* New York, W. W. Norton & Co. Inc., 1968.

Watzlawick, Paul, Janet Helmick Beavin, and Don D. Jackson. *Pragmatics of Human Communication,* New York, W. W. Norton & Co. Inc., 1967.

Index